Mahamadou Koné

Obstetrical urogenital fistulas in the hospital of Segou, Mali

Mahamadou Koné

Obstetrical urogenital fistulas in the hospital of Segou, Mali

About 56 cases

ScienciaScripts

Imprint

Any brand names and product names mentioned in this book are subject to trademark, brand or patent protection and are trademarks or registered trademarks of their respective holders. The use of brand names, product names, common names, trade names, product descriptions etc. even without a particular marking in this work is in no way to be construed to mean that such names may be regarded as unrestricted in respect of trademark and brand protection legislation and could thus be used by anyone.

Cover image: www.ingimage.com

This book is a translation from the original published under ISBN 978-620-2-28705-0.

Publisher:
Sciencia Scripts
is a trademark of
Dodo Books Indian Ocean Ltd. and OmniScriptum S.R.L publishing group

120 High Road, East Finchley, London, N2 9ED, United Kingdom
Str. Armeneasca 28/1, office 1, Chisinau MD-2012, Republic of Moldova, Europe
Printed at: see last page
ISBN: 978-620-5-90909-6

SUMMARY

DEDICATES

I dedicate this work to :

- **All women with fistula**

- **My father : Abdoulaye Koné**

I can't thank you enough.

You have always been there for us, you have always encouraged me in the direction of excellence, you have always told me that only work frees man.

Thank you for your education, I will do everything in my power to honor you.

- **My mother : Kadia Cissé**

A fighting woman that any child would have wanted as a mother.

I thank God for having you as my mother, I lack words to say thank you.

I pray to God to give us long life so that I am what you would have wanted.

- **My brother and sisters: Amadou, Rokiatou, Fatoumata, Dicko, Oumou, Alimatou, Saran, and Mariam Koné.**

You have always been there, supporting me in difficult times.

Thank you for all your support.

- **My aunt : Oumou Cissé**

You have been a mother to me, advice has never been lacking for me.

Thank you for everything you have done for us.

ACKNOWLEDGEMENTS

My sincere thanks to :

- **My country Mali**, for the quality of the education received.

My duty is to serve you with all my heart and all my strength.

- **All the teachers of the F.M.O.S**, for the quality of the teaching received.

- **To the staff of the general surgery department of the HNFS** for the good collaboration.

- **To the staff of the operating room and the intensive care unit:**

Your availability and your rigor in the work well done marked me a lot, thank you.

- **The Modibo Cissé family and Mrs. Cissé Modio Soumaré**

Throughout my medical school years, you have always been there for me, I have always felt at home. Thank you, may God give you a long life.

- **Dr. Coulibaly Mohamed**

- **Fanta Koné and Family**

- **Moussa Cissé and Family**

- **All my aunts**

- **All cousins**

- **Mamadou Koné dit Savant** and all his cyber staff in Lafiabougou

- **My childhood friends:** Aly Sacko, Boubacar Yalcoué, Gaoussou Diallo, Damis, Yacouba Sacko, Malamine Diarra.

- **My elders of the surgery department:** Dr Kamissoko A, Dr Maiga A, Dr Koné Ousmane, Dr Samaké A.

Thank you for your teaching.

- **My comrades of the F.M.O.S:** Coulibaly Lahassana, Doucouré Sidi Modibo, Traoré L, Bah Sadio, Dr Coulibaly Adama, Mallé Oumar, Koné Ladji, Traoré Moussa, Kouressi Mariam, Coulibaly Afissétou, Maiga Oumar

- **Dr Keita Mahamoudou, Dr Beye Seydina, Dr Koné Sory :**

I thank God for having benefited from your respective teachings and I pray to God to give us a long life so that I can still learn from you.

- All those who have supported me in this work from far or near, I thank you and my gratitude is without measure.

Tributes to the members of the jury

To our master and president of the jury

Professor SANOGO Zimogo Zie

- **Associate Professor of General Surgery**

- **Lecturer of semiology and surgical pathology at the F.M.O.S.**

- **Hospital practitioner at the Point G University Hospital**

- **Best surgeon of Mali award of the CNOM**

Dear Master,

We are very sensitive to the honor you have bestowed upon us by accepting to chair the jury of this thesis. We have been deeply touched by your simplicity, your modesty, your pedagogy in transmitting your knowledge.

Your availability, your great scientific culture, your qualities as a good teacher, your love of work well done, explain the esteem that all the students of the Faculty hold for you.

As a model of an exemplary surgeon, your work, both in teaching, in hospital practice and in post-graduate training, has largely contributed to the promotion of surgery in Mali.

We are convinced that you are a model of intellectual and executive for our country. Receive here dear master our sincere thanks, and our greatest respect. May God give you long life so that we can inherit your many virtues.

To our master and judge

Doctor DIAKITÉ Mamadou Lamine

- **Urological surgeon, Andrologist**

- **Hospital practitioner at the Point G University Hospital**

- **Master assistant at the F.M.O.S**

Dear Master,

We have had the pleasure of knowing you and appreciating the rigorous and hardworking man that you are.

We are very touched by your dynamism, your courage and your modesty. Your criticisms, suggestions and encouragement have been of great help in improving the quality of this work.

Allow us, dear master, to express our respect and gratitude. May God give you long life so that we can inherit your many virtues.

To our master and co-director of the thesis

Doctor SAMAKÉ Bréhima

- **Specialist in general surgery.**

- **Specialist in obstetrical vesico-vaginal fistula.**

- **Head of the general surgery department of the HNF of Ségou.**

Dear Master,

You do us a great honor by entrusting us with this work.

Your scientific approach, your availability and your frankness make you an example to follow.

You will always be our inspiration.

The clarity of your scientific reasoning, your strength of character, your technical competence, will mark us throughout our existence.

Please accept the expression of our respect and our deepest gratitude!

May God give you long life so that we may inherit your many virtues.

To our master and thesis director

Professor TEMBELY Aly Douro

- **Urological Surgeon**

- **Endo-Urologist**

- **Andrologist**

- **Specialist in extracorporeal lithotripsy**

- **International expert of the F.V.V.**

- **Head of the Urology Department of the Point G University Hospital**

- **Lecturer at the F.M.O.S**

- **Study Director of the CES/Urology in Mali**

Dear Master,

Your constant availability, your competence, your demand for a job well done, your immense human qualities have marked us forever.

The clarity of your teaching and your great scientific culture impose respect and admiration.

You are and you will be for us the example of rigor and uprightness in the exercise of the profession.

Be assured, dear master, of our deep gratitude.

May God give you long life so that we may inherit your many virtues.

ABBREVIATIONS

A.C.A.F : Association of French-speaking African Surgeons

A.F.O.A : Association for the treatment of African obstetrical fistulas.

A.M.C.F.O : Malian Association of Obstetric Fistula Surgeons. **CHU :** University Hospital Center

Cm: Centimeter

ANC: Antenatal Consultation

Cscom: Community Health Centre

Csref: Centre de santé de référence

Dr: Doctor

FO: Obstetric Fistula

A.O.F.: African obstetric fistula

F.U.G.O : Obstetrical Urogenital Fistula

VVF: Vesico-vaginal fistula

FUV : Utero-vaginal fistula

RVF: Recto-vaginal fistula

F.M.O.S : Faculty of Medicine and Odontostomatology

h : time

H.N.F.S : Nianankoro Fomba Hospital of Segou

mg: milligram

mn : minute

No.: Number

WHO: World Health Organization

NGO: Non-Governmental Organization

S.O.N.U : Emergency Obstetrical and Neonatal Care

IVU : Intravenous Urography

UCR : Retrograde Uretro-Cystography

UNFPA: United Nations Populations Fund.

I. Introduction:

Urogenital fistulas (UGFs) involve communication between a part of the urinary system (bladder, ureter, bladder neck and urethra) and a part of the genital system (uterus and vagina) and may be associated with a rectovaginal fistula[1]. These different abnormal urinary communications have been called obstetric fistulas (OF), because they are all the result of a poorly conducted or dystocic delivery, most often or in the majority of cases.

The concept of "African obstetric fistulas" encompasses several anatomical varieties including: vesico-vaginal, urethro-vaginal, utero-vaginal, uretero-vaginal, and recto-vaginal fistulas because they are most commonly encountered in Africa and have been described.

A true social and psychological tragedy, every day approximately 800 women die from complications related to pregnancy or childbirth worldwide. For every woman who dies from maternal causes, it is estimated that at least 20 suffer from maternal morbidity, one of the most severe forms of which is obstetric fistula. Two to three point five million women suffer from obstetric fistula in developing countries and 50,000 to 100,000 new cases occur each year [2].

Obstetric urogenital fistula (O.U.F.) can affect any woman or girl suffering from prolonged or obstructed labor who does not have timely access to an emergency cesarean section. It is one of the most devastating consequences of neglected childbirth and a stark example of global health inequities. Although UGF has been eliminated in industrialized countries [3], it continues to affect the poorest women and girls in developing countries, primarily in rural and remote areas.

In Mali, the maternal mortality rate is 368 per 100,000 live births according to data from the latest "Demographic and Health Survey" conducted in 2012-2013.

For every mostly preventable maternal death, 20 to 30 women survive with sequelae, one of the most serious of which is obstetric fistula [4].

Three out of five women (3/5) consulted at the Point G Urology Department suffer from VVF and treatment of VVF represents approximately 1215% of the surgical activity of this department [5].

At the hospital in Segou, it represents 3.2% of surgical activities [6].

F.U.G.O. affects young women, mostly primiparous and living in areas of difficult access.

In spite of the efforts made in prevention and the construction of health centers in our country, FUO still remains a public health problem; this is why we undertook this study to assess its management.

To carry out this work we set ourselves the following objectives:

1. General Objective:

> To study obstetrical urogenital fistulas at the Nianankoro Fomba Hospital in Segou.

2. Specific Objectives:

> Analyze the socio-demographic aspects

> Identify risk factors

> Analyze the therapeutic aspects.

II. GENERAL:

> . **Definition:** Urogenital fistulas involve communication between a part of the urinary system (bladder, ureter, bladder neck and urethra) and a part of the genital system (uterus and vagina) and may be associated with a recto-vaginal fistula. These various abnormal urinary tract communications have been termed obstetric fistulas (OF), as they are all thought to result from a poorly conducted or dystocic delivery in most or all cases.

The concept of "African obstetric fistulas" encompasses several anatomical varieties including: vesico-vaginal, urethro-vaginal, utero-vaginal, uretero-vaginal, and recto-vaginal fistulas because they are most commonly encountered in Africa and have been described.

> . **History of VFW: [7]**

> The notion of this infirmity goes back to the mists of time "if a woman has permanently leaking urine, she will lose it all her life" said Papyrus-Ebers 2000 years before Jesus Christ.

> The discovery of a vesico-vaginal fistula on the mummy of Heinheit 2050 years before Jesus Christ.

> Avicenna (1037): reports the existence of definitive bladder tearing in women married too young.

> Louis de Mercado (1597): introduces the notion of fistula.

> H-Van Roonhuyze (1663): advocates avivement and en bloc suture of the fistula.

> Pawlik (1882): proposes the catheterization of the ureters.

> Ch. Noble (1901): successfully used the mobilization of the small lip to reconstitute the urethra.

> Trendelenburg (1884): recommended the high route and use of the catgut for bladder suture.

> Fran (1894): uses for the first time the mixed approach (dissection from above, suture from below).

> L.Forgue (1904), then C.Legueu (1914): propose the transperitoneal route.

> Martius H. (1928): uses the bulbo and ischiocavernous muscles to replace the loss of substance (Martius graft).

> Christophe Walter (1679), then J.Fatios (1752): already point out the interest of bladder catheterization during labor as an important element of prevention of VVF.

> Levret (1766): to whom we owe the first description of the genu pectoral position in the surgery of the vesico-vaginal fistula!

> J. SIMS (1813-1883): created two fistula hospitals in the USA.

> Becker Brown (1859): prepares the sclerotic vagina by episiotomies, section of the flanges and Mickulicz type meching until it heals into a wide vagina.

> Maurice Collins (1861), then Duboue de Pau (1864): describe the inter-vesico-vaginal dissection (vesico-vaginal duplication).

> J.Monseur (1976): urethroplasty using the roots of the clitoris and (1980): replacement of the vagina by a sigmoidal graft.

> Abdel latifBenchekroun (1978): ileocecal continental shunt with hydraulic valve.

As can be seen, the history of VVF is in fact intertwined with the history of its treatment.

3. History of VVF management in Mali:

Surgical care for women with fistula in Mali dates back to 1906, when the Point G Hospital was created. Moreover, it is to these women that we owe the existence of the village of Point G.

This care was first provided by French military surgeons, then relayed by Malian and expatriate general surgeons, among whom we can mention Doctors ROUGERIE (Founder of the urology service), HAMAHOUI, JONCHERE, Professor Mamadou Lamine TRAORE.

From 1982 to today, the care is provided by our masters: **Professor Kalilou Ouattara** (retired since December 2014), **Professor Tembely Aly Douro** (currently Head of the Department of Urology and the Unit of management of VVF at the CHU Point G).

4. Anatomical and physiological reminders in relation to obstetric vesico-vaginal fistula:

The possibility of a fistula occurring between the bladder, cervix, urethra and the female genital organs, in this case the vagina, is essentially due to the anatomical links that connect these different organs.

First of all, they all come from the same embryological sources, which means that they have close anatomical links by their situation, being all in the pelvis, by their vascularization which comes from the same source (internal hypogastric artery), by their common sympathetic and parasympathetic innervation (hypogastric nerves and erector nerves) and finally by their kinetics, the movement of one leading to the movement of the others.

In addition, the bladder can be dragged along by the uterus and the vagina by the existence of a vesico-uterine septum and a cleavable vesico-vaginal septum. The anterior part of the bladder base responds to the vagina through the vesico-vaginal septum, the posterior part responds to the isthmus of the uterus through the vesico uterine cul-de-sac. In front, the bladder neck and the urethra are intimately linked to the vagina. It is through the vagina that the bladder rests on the perineum, in particular on the levator ani.

Before labor, pregnancy does not have much influence on the lower apparatus, because the bladder neck does not change its position, it always remains 3 cm behind the symphysis. Only the bladder capacity is decreased because of the pressure that the uterus exerts on the bladder: frequent urination.

During the work the active engagement of the presentation will transform the standards:

-Urethral lengthening of 1 to 3 cm

-The neck approaches the symphysis

-The bladder is pushed up and forward and is often bilobed. The narrowed area is more exposed to compression

In case of long dystocia, the presentation is blocked in the excavation. The cervix and trigone, immediately retro symphysial, are brought against the bony wall of the pubis and compressed. This compression constitutes a tourniquet to the circulation. Ischemic compression explains all intra pelvic lesions: fistulas and paralysis.

4.1. Anatomical reminders:

4.1.1. Female pelvis:

The normal female pelvis is characterized by well-known dimensions.

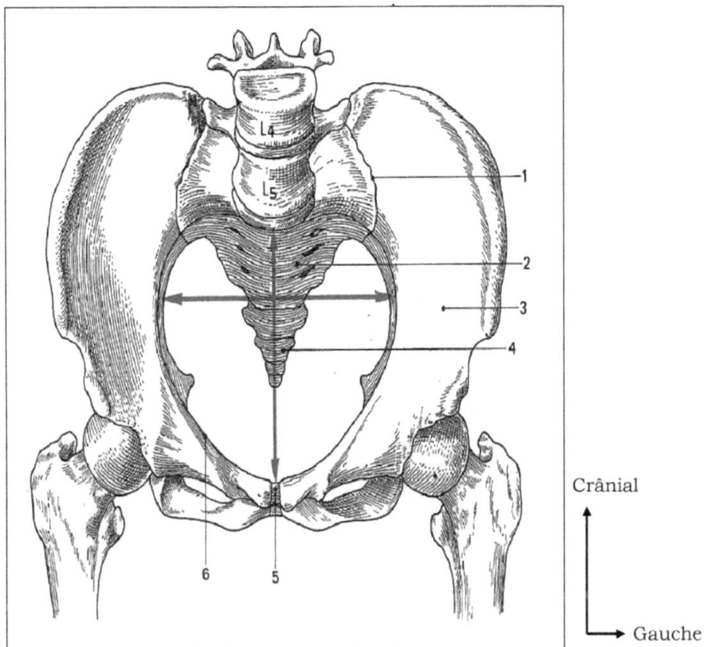

Figure 1: Female pelvis: anterosuperior view (from

FARABEUF) [8]

1- sacroiliac joint

2- Sacrum

3-Iliac eye

4-Coccyx

5- Pubic symphysis

6- Terminal line

The diameters of the upper strait are indicated by the arrows.

> **Diameters of the upper strait**

15

- Anterior - posterior diameters

- Promonto -sus pubis: 11cm

- Promonto -retro pubic: 10.5 cm

- Promonto- sub-pubic: 12 cm

- Slanting diameters: 12 cm

• Cross-sectional diameters :

- The median transverse: 13 cm

- The sacro- cotyloid : 9 cm

- **Diameters of the lower strait**

• Sub-coccyx sub-pubic diameter: 9.5 cm (11 to 12 cm in retropulsion).

• Diameter under sacro - under pubic: 11 cm.

These diameters are those of a normal pelvis. Their modification, especially their isolated or global decrease, pronounced especially those of the superior strait create a serious mechanical obstacle for the progression of the fetal mobile. This situation is known as osseous or mechanical dystocia according to the obstetrical term.

The diagnosis of dystocia must be made before labor. This implies that the expectant mother has attended prenatal consultations.

Obstetrically, women are classified into three categories:

- **Woman with normal pelvis:**

All diameters of the superior strait are normal, vaginal delivery is possible and should be allowed.

- **Woman with a borderline pelvis:**

Isolated decrease in promonto-retropubic diameter (<10.5 cm). Proof of labor is indicated.

- **Female with generally shrunken pelvis** (BGR):

Proportional decrease in overall diameters and preservation of overall pelvic morphology, cesarean section indicated.

The pelvis of adolescents corresponds to the BGR because it is immature.

Unfortunately, they are very often married at an early age in our context and therefore exposed to mechanical dystocia due to obstetric vesicovaginal fistula.

However, in our context, even women with a normal pelvis are not spared from dystocia because, in addition to mechanical dystocia, they can be victims of dynamic dystocia, especially since the rate of medicalized delivery is very low.

4.1.2. Relationship between the bladder and the pelvic organs :

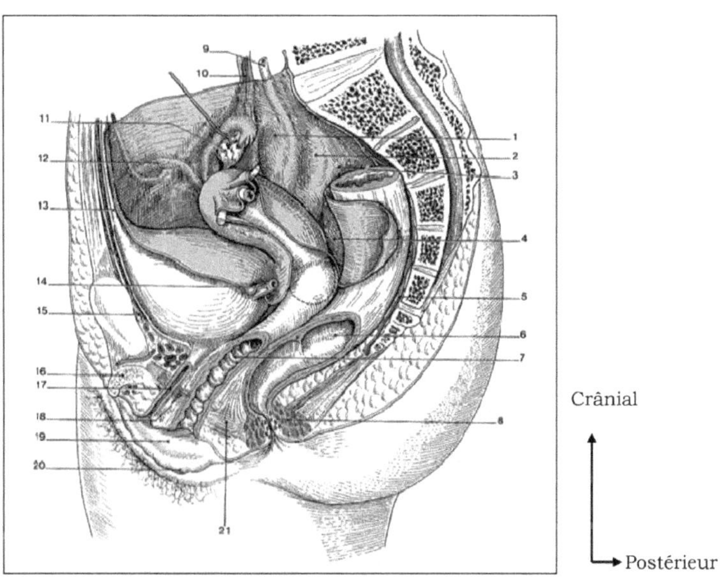

Figure 2: Paramedian sagittal section of the female pelvis after P. KAMINA [9]

1- ovarian dimple	11- Ovary
2- infra ovarian dimple	12- Round ligament
3- Recto uterine fold	13-Ouraque
4- Recto uterine cul de sac	14-Left ureter
5- a .median sacral	15- Pre-bladder space
6- Rectum	16- Clitoris
7- Vagina	17- Urethra
8- m. of the external sphincter of the anus	18- m. external sphincter of the urethra

9- Right ureter   19- Small lip

10- Suspensory ligament of the ovary   20- Large lip

21- pectineal tendon center

It is well known that the urinary tract and the genital organs emanate from the same embryonic tissues and that they have the same sources of vascularization and innervation and that their kinetics are closely linked.

Their vascularization comes mainly from branches of the inferior hypogastric (inferior vesical artery), uterine artery (vesical branches), pudendal artery (anterior vesical artery), permeable part of the umbilical artery and obturator artery (superior vesical arteries).

The venous circuit, as we know, forms the plexus of Santorini on the anterior surface of the bladder, and the venous branches formed - vesical veins, uterine veins - then join the internal hypogastric (iliac) veins.

The lymphatic pathways go to the internal iliac nodes, obturator nodes, and then to the external iliac nodes or primitive iliac nodes.

Innervation is provided by the 3rd and 4th sacral nerves and especially by the hypogastric plexus (mixed nerves).

The bladder is connected to the organs of the lesser pelvis through the bladder space filled with connective tissue, which is limited by fibrous-serous formations: the pelvic peritoneum above, the umbilical-pre-vesical fascia in front and behind, the anterior wall of the vagina below and behind, the posterior face of the pubic symphysis, which separates it from the anterior face of the bladder, creating the space called the space of Retzius.

This said, the posterior surface of the empty bladder serves as a support for the body of the uterus. With a full bladder, the ascension of the uterus causes the base of the bladder to come into contact with the isthmus of the uterus via the peritoneum. The peritoneum, after having lined the posterior superior surface of the bladder, curves into a cul de sac and then covers the anteroinferior surface of the uterine body. Under the vesico-uterine peritoneal cul de sac is the vesico-uterine septum. The relationship with the vagina is such that the bladder rests essentially on its anterior wall.

4.2 Physiological reminders :

4.2.1. Normal delivery:

Delivery is the set of phenomena that result in the exit of the fetus and its appendages from the maternal genital tract, once the pregnancy has reached the term of 37 to 42 weeks of amenorrhea.

These phenomena are governed by the adaptation of the dimensions of the fetal diameters, those of the fetal head in particular, to that of the maternal pelvis and the soft parts. Coupled with uterine contractions, they allow the fetus to cross the birth canal.

The course of the delivery includes 3 phases:

- effacement and dilation of the uterine cervix;

- expulsion or exit of the fetus from the genital tract;

- the exit of the placenta (delivery).

The first period is marked by the appearance of uterine contractions (onset of labor) and its consequences are on :

- The uterus itself with formation and appearance of the lower segment, effacement and dilation of the cervix;

- The lower pole of the egg leading to the rupture and cleavage of the membranes (amnion and chorion);

- The fetal mobile: the contractions push the fetus downwards to make it cross the different levels of the pelvi-genital tract in three stages: - The engagement which corresponds to the crossing of the superior strait with orientation and reduction of the presentation, - The descent and the rotation

- The release corresponds to the crossing of the lower strait. The whole of this progression is called the mechanical phenomena of childbirth. This first phase is the longest of the delivery, it lasts on average 7-10 hours in primiparous women and 3-6 hours in multiparous women.

The second period includes 2 phases:

- The completion of the descent and rotation of the presentation,

- The expulsion itself with a sum of mechanical phenomena (release) including the crossing of the inferior osteomalacic strait and the crossing of the pelvi-perineal floor.

The duration of this period is 1-2 hours on average in primiparous women. A labor period longer than 18 hours is harmful to the mother and even more so to the child, hence the importance of monitoring the labor.

The set of abnormalities that can hinder the normal progress of the delivery is called a dystocia. It can be either abnormalities of uterine contraction and cervical dilation: this is called dynamic dystocia or poor accommodation of the fetus to the maternal pelvis: this is called mechanical dystocia.

Sometimes there is a link between these two anomalies, with dynamic dystocia occurring over an underlying mechanical dystocia.

4.2.2. Anatomical changes of the bladder during gestation: These are topographical changes: when the presentation is not engaged, pregnancy does not have much influence on the lower urinary tract because the bladder neck remains 3 cm from the pubic symphysis, only the bladder capacity is reduced due to the compression of the uterus on the bladder.

Active engagement will transform these norms:

- the urethra lengthens by 1-3cm,

- the bladder neck moves closer to the pubic symphysis, - the bladder is pushed up and forward.

It is easy to understand that excessive stretching of the ligaments and fascias during dystocia or obstetrical maneuvers causes disorders with definitive and innumerable consequences: the cervix and trigone, immediately retro-symphysial, are brought against the bony wall of the pubis and compressed. This compression constitutes a tourniquet to the blood circulation and explains all the intra pelvic ischemic lesions.

5. Etio-pathogenesis:

We will only mention the African obstetric fistula (A.O.F.).

F.O.A. is almost always the consequence of a difficult and prolonged delivery in a place generally lacking adequate technical facilities and especially qualified personnel. In short, it is a dystocic, dynamic or anatomic delivery. The labor has started, the head of the fetus is now blocked in the small pelvis.

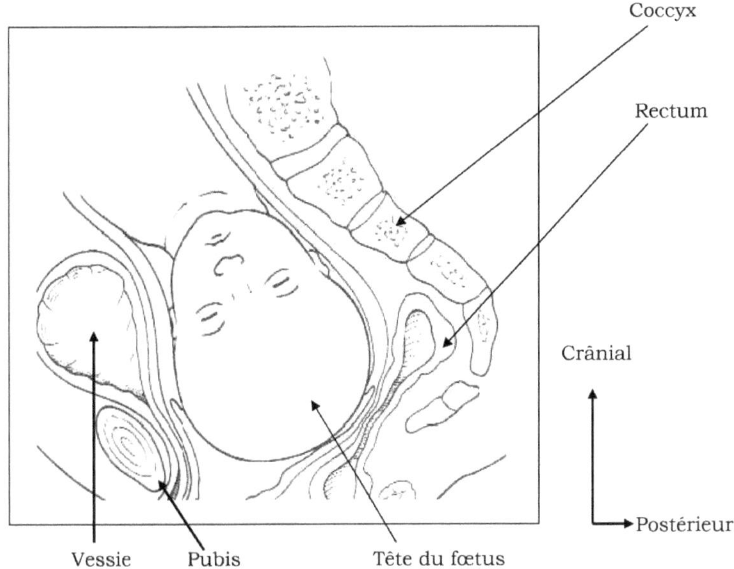

Figure 3 [7]: Mother's pelvis and fetus during delivery.

Prolonged compression of the bladder wall between the presentation and the posterior edge of the pubic symphysis causes ischemia followed by more or less extensive necrosis of the organs of the lesser pelvis: uterine cervix, vesico-vaginal septum, bladder neck, rectum etc.

However, all authors agree that ischemic necrosis of the pelvic organs followed by eschar fall at 3-4 weeks is the main mechanism of fistula installation. However, an overly expeditious delivery may tear the cervix to the bladder base, resulting in VF.

According to MONSEUR, prolonged bladder distension is the determining factor in the necrosis of the bladder wall, especially since it is aggravated by the fact that traditional birth attendants force-feed their parturients with water. The bladder wall is subjected to two opposing forces, that of the blocked presentation and the hydraulic pressure of the retained urine.

Other factors favoring the occurrence of obstetric bladder fistula

They are of 3 types: medical, socio-cultural and economic.

5.1. Medical:

22

This is the low obstetrical coverage.

Our statistics in this area are as follows:

1 doctor for 40000 inhabitants

1 specialist doctor for 200 to 300,000 inhabitants

oAbout 45-50 gynecologists - midwives

o6 urological surgeons

o600 midwives

o Add to this the lack of infrastructure.

5.2. Sociocultural:

To this catastrophic situation we must add certain harmful practices such as genital mutilation and early marriages, which are commonplace in our context, all against a background of poverty and widespread illiteracy.

5.3. Economic:

Widespread poverty.

6. Anatomy and pathology:

Three aspects must be taken into account: the location of the fistula, the state of the tissues, the associated lesions

6.1. Fistula site:

On this plan 4 groups are to be retained

6.1.1. Retro trigonal (high iatrogenic): They communicate the posterior aspect of the bladder with the vaginal stump and sit distant from the ureteral meatus and urethral meatus.

6.1.2. Trigonal: They are located near the ureteral meatus which can be taken during the repair.

6.1.3. Cervical: The bladder neck and sphincters are affected; continence is compromised even after cure of the V.F.

6.1.4. Cervical - urethral: Sit on the cervix and urethra which can be seriously damaged

6. 2. Tissue condition:

The anatomical description is not sufficient to judge the severity of the fistula.

To this must be added certain important details such as trophicity, which assesses the quality and vitality of the tissues, and fibrosis, which provides information on the state of the vagina

Three degrees of trophicity are noted:

> Trophicity good

Soft, thick, well-vascularized and non-adherent tissues

> Medium trophy

Macroscopically normal thinned tissues appearing cleavable

> Poor trophicity

Rigid, thinned tissues intimately adherent to the pubic periosteum

Three degrees of fibrosis are noted:

> Absent fibrosis: quasi-normal vagina

> Medium fibrosis: requires simple debridement.

> Important fibrosis: important losses of substance after excision to be filled.

> **.3. Associated lesions:**

During the fistula, other organs can present important lesions which can be of the following types

6.3.1. Gynaecological :

6.3.1.1. At the level of the uterus: the uterus is of normal volume. It is immobile on traction because of the extension of the fibrosis to the ligaments of MACKENRODT. This makes it difficult to expose the anterior vaginal wall and therefore the fistula. The cervix may be healthy, or it may be short and buried in the mass of sclerosis, or it may be shredded, with disappearance of the cul de sacs.

It may be stenotic or remodeled and deformed at the anterior lip. A fixed uterine reversion may be observed. Urine flow at the level of a scar indicates the existence of a vesico uterine fistula. This fistula is in contact with a torn cervix and is prone to infection.

Tubal infertility, endometritis, chronic salpingitis, amenorrhea and dysovulations can be found.

6.3.1.2. In the vagina: the atresic vagina is invaded by a rigid fibrosis that often only allows the passage of a single finger. This fibrosis makes examination of the fistula difficult even under general anesthesia. Sexual intercourse is impossible.

On the posterior surface, an arched, semi-lunar frontal flange can also be seen. This flange is prolonged posteriorly, sharp, docking the posterior lip of the uterine cervix and erasing the fornix.

Retractable flanges can make it impossible to examine the cervix valve even under general anesthesia. The cervix is literally pushed into a sort of vaginal backbone that prevents the evacuation of menses (hematocolpos). We then witness an impressive atresia of the vagina. Its mucous membrane is smooth, whitish and varnished. It is extremely sensitive to touch. All the normal folds have disappeared.

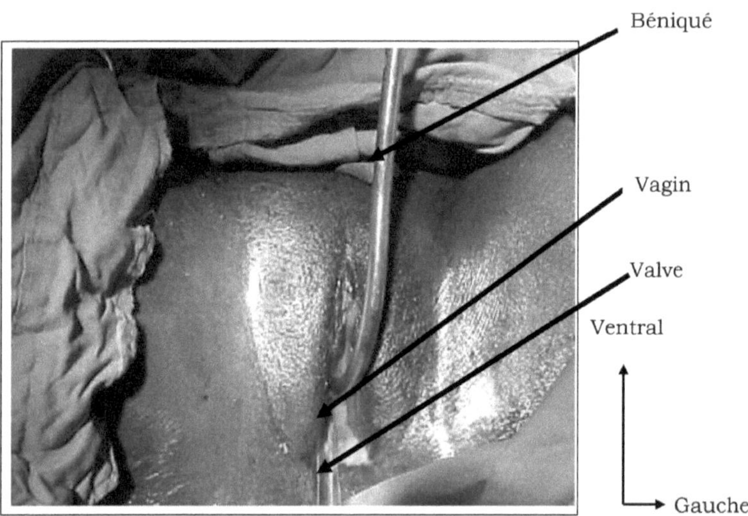

Image from the urology department of the Point G University Hospital: Vaginal atresia preventing examination of the vagina.

6.3.1.3. At the level of the vulva:

The vulva is often the site of exulcerated and superinfected condylomas and vegetations

6.3.1.4. At the level of the perineum:

They are easily diagnosed. They are most often sequelae of a complete tear (type II) with rupture of the anal sphincter ring or complicated tears (type III) with opening and extension of the anal canal and the recto vaginal septum. The central fibrous core of the perineum having burst, only the posterior anal half-circumference remains intact. Associated type II: low rectovaginal lesions only involve the lower third of the vagina. They may be single or multiple with difficult access due to a posterior vaginal wall flange. This flange forms a recess where the recto vaginal fistula is hidden. It can also be a question of lesions that result from a complete or complicated rupture of the perineum. The repair of this rupture, most often carried out in poor conditions on poorly cleansed tissues, results in a more or less complete disunion. This leads to the formation of cutaneous-mucosal bridges that are more or less synechial.

Certain traditional practices such as infibulation and excision are responsible for expulsion dystocia, exposing the perineum to tears.

6.3.2. Digestive :

In the rectum: These are traumatic lesions related to ischemia by prolonged compression. These lesions lead to secondary opening by the fall of eschar. They can be high and punctiform, and may be unrecognized at the bottom of an atresic vagina. This hole only lets out a little gas and or some liquid stools. Elsewhere, they can be high and giant, reaching several centimeters in diameter, creating a real colostomy.

They may be lesions of sphincter rupture and lesions of the recto-vaginal septum of varying height. Sometimes flanges in the posterior wall of the vagina can mask the lesions and thus they go unnoticed during the examination.

7. Classification:

Several types of classifications have been proposed by different authors.

Among them we can mention :

7.1. HAMLIN and NICHOLSON classification:

It divides fistulas into 6 groups according to anatomical and clinical location:

- Simple F.V.V,

- Simple F.R.V.'s,

- Simple urethrovaginal fistulas,

- The high F.R.V.'s,

- Vesico uterine fistulas,

- Complex urinary fistulas associating vesico-urethral-cervical lesions.

7.2. The COUVELAIRE classification:

It classifies fistulas into 2 major groups: pure retro-trigonal fistulas and fistulas in which there are :

- A sclerosis

- A proximity of the ureteral meatus

- A destruction of the bladder neck

- Reduced bladder capacity

- Partial or total destruction of the urethra.

7.3. BENCHEKROUN's classification:

It essentially distinguishes 3 types of fistulas:

Type I - trigono - cervical - urethral transection,

Type II - cervico-urethral destruction,

Type III - simple cervical-urethral fistula

7.4. Classification of LUGANE P. M, Leo J.P.:

She divides fistulas into 3 groups:

- Retro trigonal F.V.V.'s

- trigonal F.V.V.'s,

- Cervico-vaginal fistulas with detrusor involvement,

- Cervico-urethral fistulas with damage to the urethra and bladder sphincter.

7.5. The classification of A. MENSAH et al. :

It divides fistulas into 3 classes:

> **simple fistulas:**

They have the following characteristics:

> Away from the ureteral orifices.

> Urethra unharmed.

> No peri-fistula sclerosis.

Treatment by the vaginal route almost always results in a cure after the first operation.

> **complex fistulas:** Characterized by:

> Destroyed bladder neck

> Partial or total damage to the urethra.

> Limited perifistulous sclerosis

> It is possible to perform a vaginal cure at the cost of almost systematic urinary incontinence.

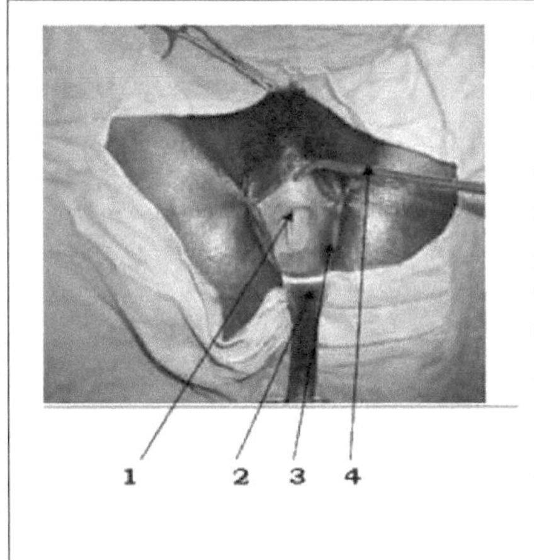
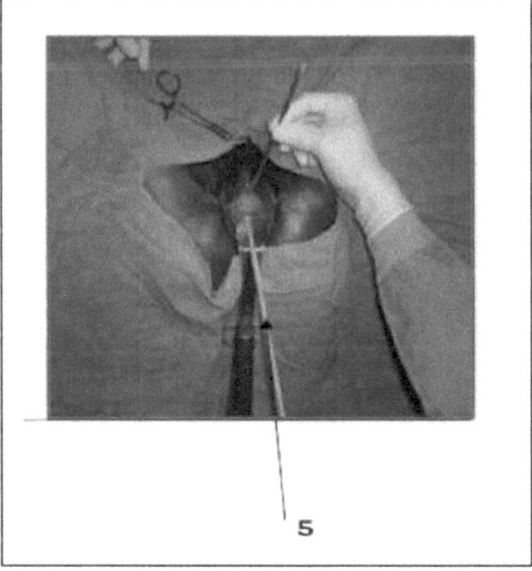

Images from the urology department of the Point G University Hospital:
simple fistulas

1-orifice of the fistula

2-valve

3-lip sutured to the thigh

4-benched

5-trans-urethral bladder probe

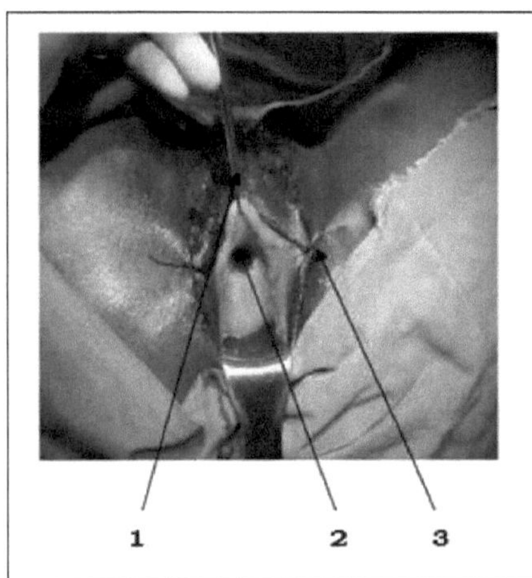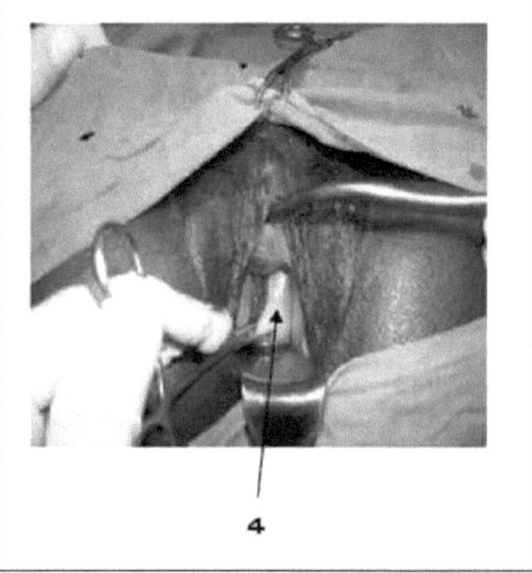

Images from the urology department of the Point G University Hospital: complex fistulas

1-dissecting   forceps4-cystocele

2-orifice of the fistula

3-lip sutured to the thigh

> **Complicated fistulas or "African" VVF**

Characterized by:

> Real urogenital and perineal decay

> Bladder neck and urethra. Destroys very extensive fistulous peri-fistula sclerosis, which can obstruct one or both ureteral meatus.

> Very difficult cure.

7.6. The A.F.O.A. (Association for the Treatment of African Obstetric Fistulas) classification, derived from the classification of Maurice CAMEY and L. FALANDRY:

The F.V.V. are classified in 3 main groups.

Simple F.V.V.'s:

Located on the posterior aspect of the bladder, at a distance from the neck, in healthy and flexible tissue, less than 3 cm in size.

Depending on the location of the fistula, they are divided into:

- High F.V.V. near the cervix;

- F.V.V. Low, near the bladder neck ;

- Middle F.V.V., in the middle of the vesico-vaginal septum.

Depending on the size of the breach, a distinction is made between:

- F.V.V. punctiform, difficult to visualize,

- The destruction of the vesico-vaginal partition admitting at least two or three fingers, allowing then the intra vesical touch, here there is no sclerosis of the healthy tissues

Complex F.V.V. :

Which include:

- The F.V.V. of the trigono - Cervico - urethral region respecting the continuity of the anterior wall of the bladder with the anterior wall of the cervix and the urethra.

- Fistulas that do not involve either the bladder neck or the urethra but have already been operated on (second hand fistulas or after several attempts at cure).

Severe VF:

Partial or total destruction of the urethra, of the bladder neck with moderate sclerosis, an obstructed urethra (blind) should be noted here.

Note that the sclerosis can be important (cardboard vagina), consequence of the invasion of the urogenital tract by a scleroinfectious process.

7.7. Classification of the urology service of the Point G University Hospital (Pr. Kalilou Ouattara et al.):

7.7.1. Depending on the environment:

Three situations are possible:

A) Fistula on soft vagina,

B) Fistula on vaginal sclerosis (bridges, stenosis or vaginal atresia),

C) FVV + (Perineal tear I, II, III degree, FRV).

7.7.2. According to the anatomical location:

Type I: Vesico-vaginal septum fistula:

• The fistula is located in the middle of the vesico-vaginal septum sparing both the vesical and uterine cervixes.

• The fistula is small, medium, large or wide

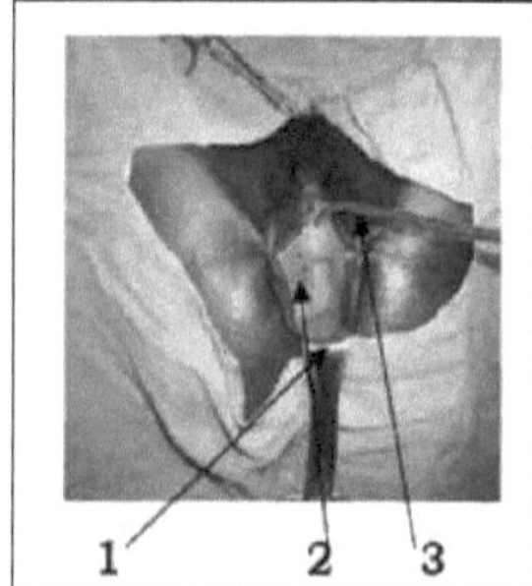
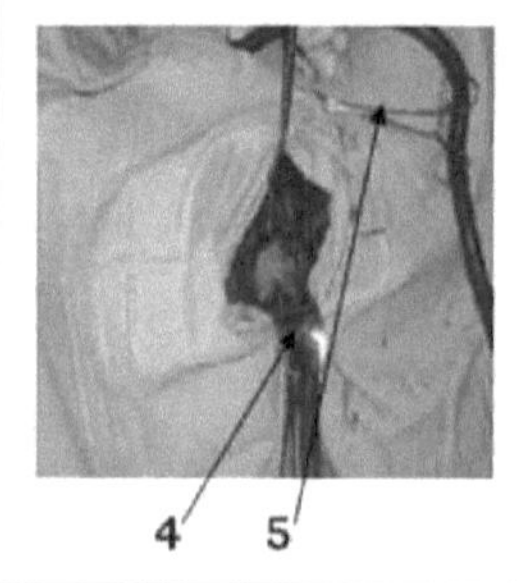
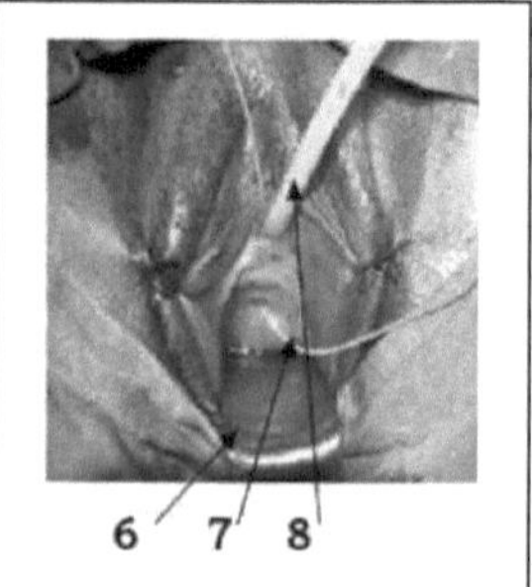

Images from the Urology Department of Point G University Hospital: 1-valve vesico-vaginal septum fistulas

2-orifice of the fistula

3-benched

4-valve

5-field clamp

6-valve

7-tubing

8-trans-urethral bladder probe

Type II: Cervical fistulas (vesico-cervical-urethro-vaginal fistulas):

• The fistula is located on the vesico-cervico-urethral segment:

Type IIA: Without destruction of the urethra

Type IIAa: cervico-urethro-vaginal

Type IIAb: Partial cervical-urethral disinsertion Type IIAc: Total cervical-

urethral disinsertion Type IIB: With destruction of the urethra.

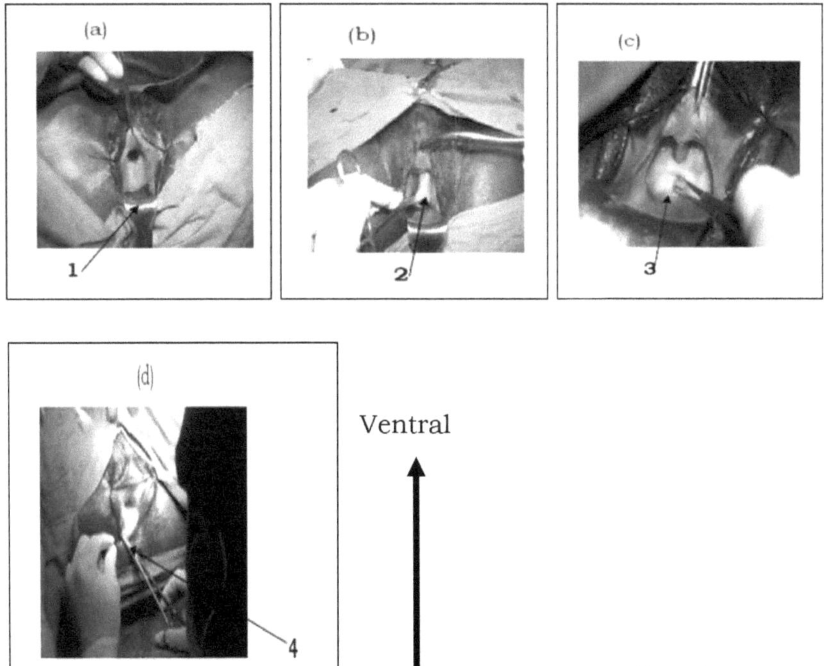

Images from the urology department of the Point G University Hospital: vesico-cervical-urethral fistulas **1-valve** 2- cervix

4-needle holder clip

Type III: Trigono-cervico-utero-vaginal fistula:

- The fistula involves the bladder trigone and the cervix

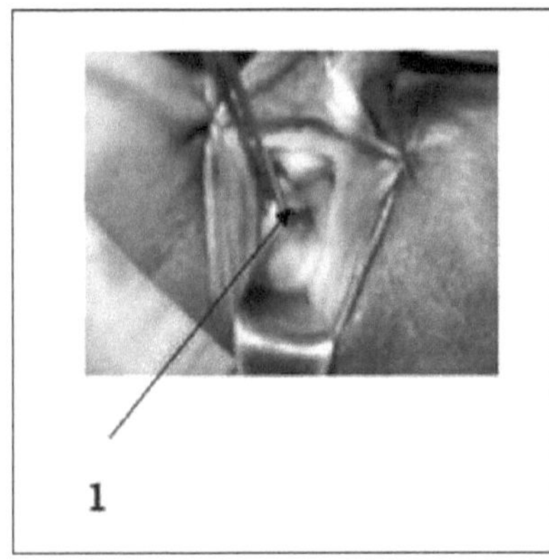
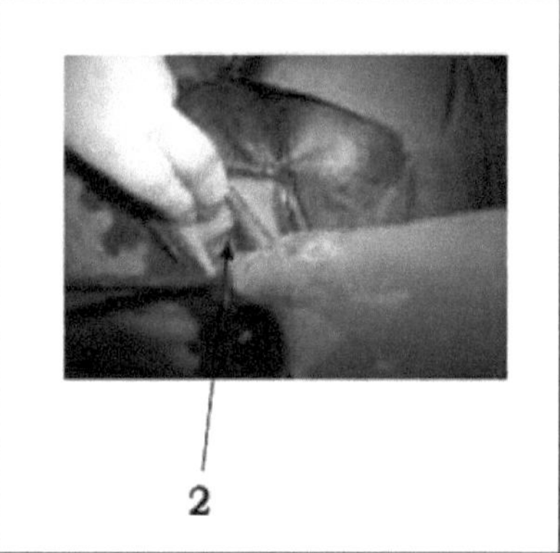

Images from the urology department of the Point G University Hospital:

Trigono-cervical-utero-vaginal fistula 1-orifice of the fistula 2- orifice of the fistula

Type IV: Complex Fistulas (Mixed):

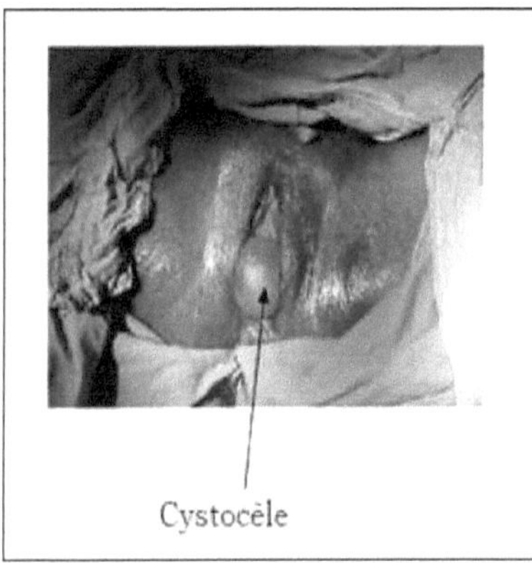

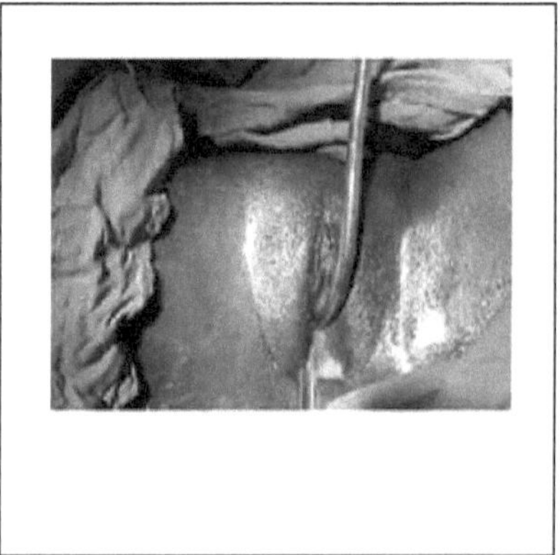

Images from the Urology Department of the Point G University Hospital:

Complex Fistulas (Mixed)

Type V : High fistulas (retrotrigonal)

-vesicovaginal

* vesico-cervico-uterine

* vesico-uterine

-Urethro-vaginal

8. Diagnosis:

8.1. Positive diagnosis:

The diagnosis of vesico-vaginal fistula is based primarily on the data of the interview and physical examination.

8.1.1. Interrogation:

It provides information on the patient's age; the circumstances of the onset of urinary incontinence.

Classically, it is a young woman of childbearing age who, in a consultation, smells urine with a characteristic ammoniacal odor, making her socially undesirable, in the aftermath of a dystocic delivery. The major sign is the uncontrolled flow of urine (urinary incontinence). This urinary incontinence is either :

-       Total.

-       Partial (with retained micturition).

-       Intermittent, more pronounced standing up (low fistula) or lying down (high fistula).

Other signs: amenorrhea, dysmenorrhea, cyclic hematuria, reflecting Youssef's triad (vesico-uterine fistula), neurological disorders, etc.

8.1.2. Physical examination:

It is performed on a patient in a gynecological position, in a spacious, well-lit room. It sometimes requires the assistance of the anesthesiologist.

> **Upon inspection:**

Ulcerations of the vulva, perineum and inner thighs due to the corrosive effect of urine attract attention.

> **Placement of a vaginal valve:**

It often allows to notice an inflammation of the anterior aspect of the vagina, to locate the fistulous orifice either directly or by the urine flow.

In the case of small fistulas lying behind folds of the vaginal mucosa, instillation of dye into the bladder (e.g. methylene blue) allows the site to be identified. A leakage of dye through the uterine cervix indicates a vesico uterine fistula.

> **The vaginal touch:**

This often allows the diagnosis to be made; the finger that touches can access the vaginal cavity in cases of great loss of substance.

8.1.3. Additional examinations:

> **Cystoscopy:**

It is of great help because it can locate the fistulous orifice and determine its relationship with the bladder neck and ureteral orifices.

The simultaneous injection of intravenous indigo carmine allows at the same time to verify the absence of lesion on the ureters. The mutilation of a ureteral meatus suspects a lesion on the corresponding ureter; it also allows to catheterize the ureters preoperatively. Cystoscopy is not feasible in large dilapidations.

> **Intravenous urography (IVU) with cystography film:**

It is essential because it allows the state of the upper urinary tract to be assessed and any ureteral lesions to be shown. The % cystogram allows to visualize most often the vesico-vaginal communication with opacification of the vagina.

The same image can show a vesico - uterine communication if it exists.

> **Retrograde Uretro Cystography (RUC):**

It should be performed when the cystography is not satisfactory to identify the path of small fistulas.

> **Ultrasound:**

It allows to appreciate the impact of the lesions on the upper urinary tract.

8.2. Differential diagnosis:

It can occur with stress incontinence, sometimes residual after "successful" surgical treatment of a V.V.F. where the loss of urine can cause discomfort close to that caused by the initial lesions. In some cases, one may wonder if it is not a residual fistula hidden in a scar fold.

Urethro-vaginal fistulas, although it is known that they can be associated with VVF, are characterized by a bladder methylene blue test and negative cystoscopy, and a late positive intravenous indigo carmine blue test, the equivocation will be removed. In all cases the diagnosis cannot be limited to the affirmation of the fistula, but must be based on a precise quantitative and qualitative description of the lesions, on the basis of a typological classification which will indicate the type of operation to be performed.

9. Treatment of vesico-vaginal fistula:

9.1. Goals:

- Restore bladder seal

- Restore continence,

- Prevent recurrence by iterative cesarean sections,

- To allow the woman to regain a normal sexual life and her ability to procreate.

- Ensure social and economic reintegration

This treatment will be curative if the above-mentioned objectives are achieved and palliative in cases where closure of the AVF is impossible, leaving the only recourse to urinary diversion

9.2. Preventive treatment:

Prevention of obstetric fistula involves:

- Information, sensitization and education of the population on the harms of early marriage;

- Improving health coverage;

- Better organization of the evacuation reference system

- Proper care of the pregnant woman (prenatal consultation, medically assisted delivery)

- Bladder catheterization during labor;

- Prophylactic caesarean section for patients who have had a fistula cure

- Family planning.

9.3. Curative treatment:

The fistula is curable in 90% of cases when it is simple and in 60% of cases when it is complex.

To ensure the lasting success of the operation, at least two weeks of postoperative care is required.

Psychological follow-up is important to treat the emotional trauma and to facilitate the social reintegration of patients

9.3.1. Means and Methods :

9.3.1.1. Medical means:

Its objective is to prepare the patient for surgery by treating a probable urogenital infection, anemia, parasitosis, constipation or diarrhea, preparing the operating field, counseling, after an assessment of the field and an operability assessment.

9.3.1.2. Surgical means:

9.3.1.2.1. General principles:

They were very well stated by R. COUVELAIRE: "see well, split well, face the surfaces well, drain the urine well", and to this should be added: do everything possible to succeed at the first attempt, because, even if the residual fistula is often less important than the original fistula, each operation carries an additional risk of devascularization and sclerosis of the tissues.

To see well, the best approach must be chosen according to the location of the fistula.

The vaginal route, which is the most commonly used, can be hampered by sclerosis, which narrows the vagina, prevents the installation of the valve and blocks access to the fistula.

Episiotomies are then necessary.

Anesthesia must allow to operate as long as necessary and in all positions, to carry out a sometimes complex operation. Unfortunately, local conditions are not always optimal and the basic anesthesia is usually spinal anesthesia, which the buvivacaine-Fintanyl association would allow to prolong as much as possible.

Beyond that, some teams only have at their disposal IV Ketamine, which, if well handled, can prolong the intervention by an hour or two.

The operation is not performed during menstruation, and any oral contraception, which is rare in these countries, is stopped.

As for the date of intervention, most of our women with fistula were examined months or years after their occurrence and the problem of early intervention did not arise. Nevertheless, without going as far as the very long delays, our attitude has tended until now to join the classic opinion of waiting three (3) months after the date of delivery.

Whenever possible, it is important not to wait any longer in order to avoid the evolution of the sclerosis.

9.3.1.2.2. Routes of approach and position:

Three approaches are possible: vaginal in dorsal or ventral position, extra or trans-peritoneal abdominal, and a mixed approach combining the two approaches. A posterior approach with coccygeal resection must be added for the treatment of certain rectal fistulas.

> **The vaginal route:**

This is the most frequently used procedure and there is no lack of arguments in its favor. It gives direct access to lesions of the cervix and urethra, which are frequent and often extensive.

It exposes the areas where the tissues used for the interpositions between the bladder and vaginal sutures will be taken. The MARTIUS graft with or without skin and the roots of the clitoris are taken from the labia majora, the rectus internus muscle (also with or without skin), from the inner side of the thigh. Finally, it involves the least risk.

J **The dorsal position:** is the most classic position and must be chosen whenever a complementary abdominal approach can be envisaged.

In order to properly expose the lesions, the buttocks must be very prominent and for bladder lesions, the slope must be very pronounced. This brings the anterior vaginal wall practically perpendicular to the operator's view. It is very important to be well lit

It may happen that the bladder wall herniates through the fistula. This protrusion must then be reduced by a bladder tamponade, which must not be forgotten to be removed during the bladder suture.

J **Prone position:**

Very classical, it has the great advantage of giving a direct view on the lesions, of spontaneously reducing the possible bladder protrusion for the fistula.

However, there is a disadvantage: the compression of the intestinal coils on the table top, which hinders respiratory movements.

> **The abdominal route:**

This is obviously the route of choice when treating a high vesico-uterine or vesico-cervical uterine fistula (with the ureteral lesion that is sometimes associated with them).

However, it is not well adapted to extensive urethral lesions and when an upper urethral plasty program is considered, access to the vulva must be provided.

The infectious risk of the tract, especially when the peritoneum is open, must be taken into account if the asepsis of the operating room is not adequately ensured.

> **The mixed abdominal-perineal route:**

It may happen that the location and character of the fistula requires a mixed approach, such as dissection of the vaginal orifice from below, dissection and closure of the bladder from above, and then closure of the vagina, after interposition of MARTIUS from below. The thighs, which are very flexed on the abdomen during the perineal time, must be able to be extended without any fault of asepsis during the abdominal time.

9.3.2. Surgical techniques and indications:

9.3.2.1. Cure of simple bladder fistulas:

By definition, these are fistulas located on the posterior aspect of the bladder, at a distance from the neck and trigone, and the ureteral orifices are far away. They will not be catheterized. Sclerosis is usually modest. Small trigonal fistulas can be included in this group, but prior cystoscopic verification of the ureteral orifices is recommended.

A benique 40 or a Foley CH18 catheter easily penetrates the bladder.

It is perceived by the fistula. It is important to make sure that there are no multiple fistulas.

Episiotomies are not necessarily the rule in this type of fistula or at least they will be short and easily sutured. The introduction of the weighted valve is not a problem.

Simple bladder fistulas are the easiest to treat and we will use this as a model to describe the basic surgical technique, the principles of which will be assumed to be known for the treatment of complicated fistulas.

This technique essentially consists of 3 steps: **Exposure, incision and cleavage:**

- **Exhibition:**

- Fixation of the lips with non-absorbable 00 thread

- Additional digital exploration

- Introduction of the valve

- Location of the F.V.V. with a benique if it is visible

- Bladder catheterization and methylene blue test

Introduction of a CH18 or 20 Foley catheter through the fistula.

Traction on the F.V.V. by the Foley probe (or by 4 wires)

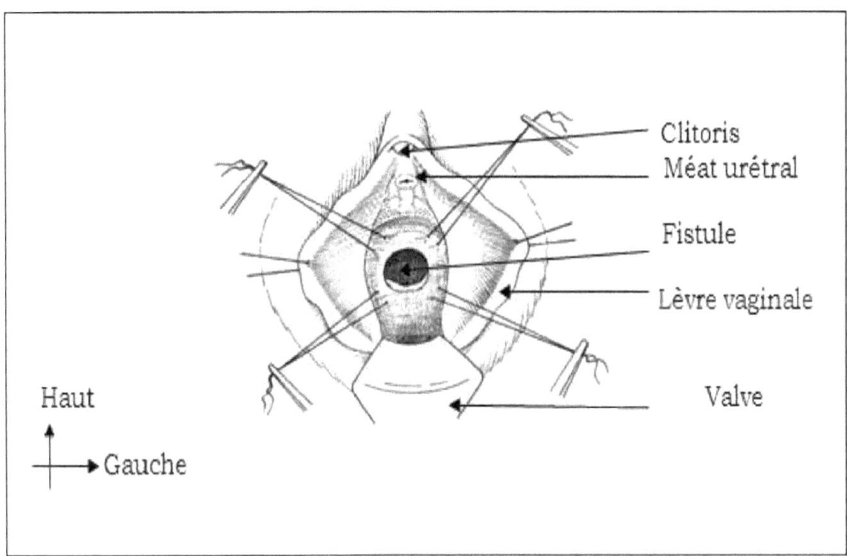

Figure 4 [7]: Fistula exposure

> **Incision:**

A circular incision, starting where access is easiest, is made at the bladder-vagina junction at the level of the fistula. If the fistula is very small, two small transverse incisions on either side of the fistula can be used.

Some small transverse incisions can help (small fistula)

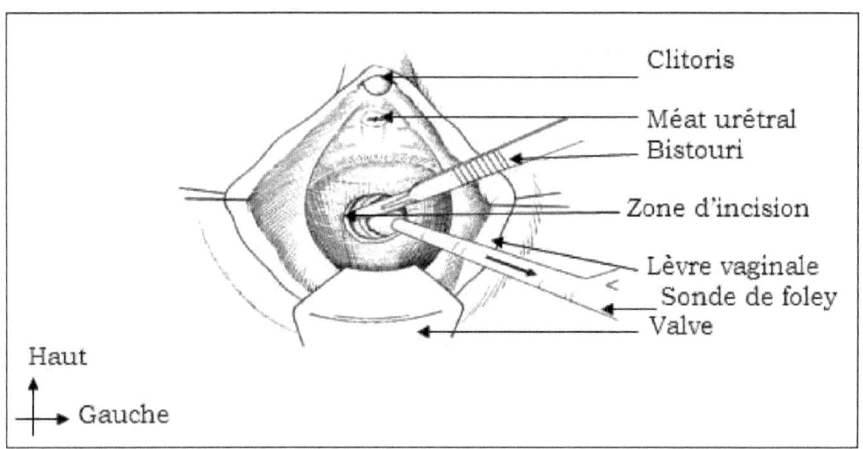

Figure 5 [7] : Incision of the bladder-vagina junction

> **Cleavage:**

With the flat scissors on the side of the curve, find the cleavage between the bladder and the vagina, keeping the entire thickness of the vaginal wall. Scissors well bent on the plane are particularly useful here.

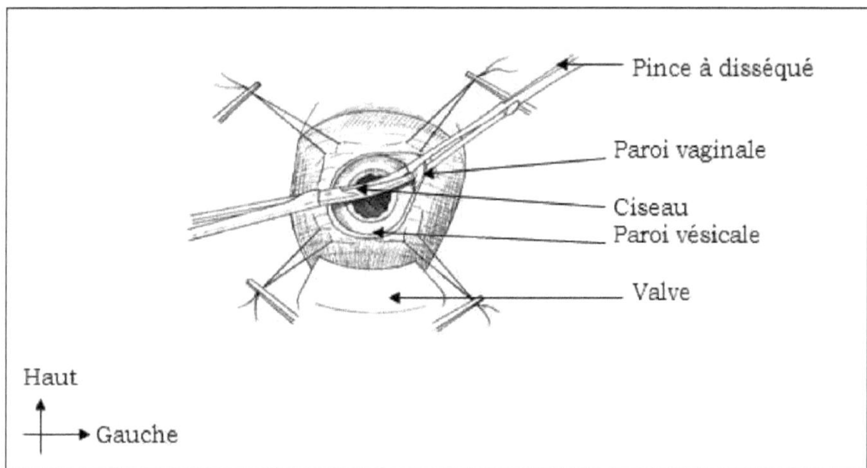

Figure 6 [7]: Cleavage between bladder and vagina

> **Bladder Suture:**

The suture of the bladder is performed in a plane of separate stitches taking well the muscle and the sub-mucosa, taking the least possible mucosa, which must not herniate.

These stitches must be close enough to ensure a seal, but not too close to avoid ischemia. Similarly, the stitches must be tightened to ensure a good fit but not to cut the tissue.

The vertical or horizontal direction of the suture is not important, but its choice must allow easy suturing of the bladder and later of the vagina.

Several nearby fistulas will be combined into one.

> **Leakage test :**

A CH18 Foley catheter is inserted through the urethra and a leakage test with blue-stained serum is performed. The sometimes reduced bladder capacity must be taken into account and overpressure must be avoided. Otherwise, any leakage requires an additional suture, unless it occurs through the needle holes. This may eventually lead to an interposition.

> **Vaginal Suture:**

The suture of the vagina is also performed in a separate stitch plane. The direction of the suture is not important. It is important that the suture is performed without traction, but if possible, it should not correspond to the bladder suture line.

It must allow the dead space between the bladder and the vagina to be erased and must face the vagina well. For this, U-shaped or BLAIRE DONATI type stitches are effective.

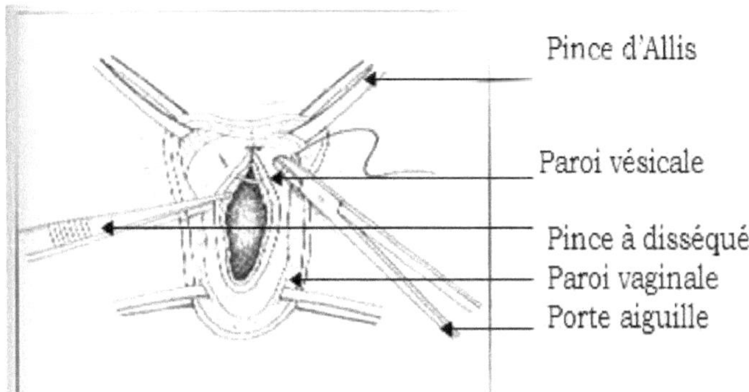

Figure 7 [7]: Suture of the bladder

> **The Operation of CHASSAR- MOIR:**

It is in fact a refinement of the original technique described in 1852 by MARIONS SIMS

> **Technical:**

The patient is placed in the waist position described above. A catheter is placed in the bladder. Four ALLIS forceps, placed in a diamond pattern around the fistula, grasp the vagina and lower it to the vulva; a balloon catheter may be placed in the bladder through the fistula opening. Pulling on the catheter would produce the same effect.

The different operating times are :

> ƒ **Vertical incision of the vagina: (fig.8)**

The incision starts 1 cm above the fistula opening, goes around the opening and ends 1 cm below it.

S **Vesico-vaginal detachment: (fig.9)**

It is not very extensive, the objective being to avoid any dead space between the vesicovaginal wall and the vagina. A 10 to 15 mm detachment around the fistula is generally sufficient and will allow a good contact with the vaginal wall.

S **Closure of the bladder outlet: (fig.10)**

It is performed in one or two planes, preferably extra mucosal, in separate stitches with 3/0 Vicryl.

S **Checking the bladder seal: (fig.11)**

It is done by injecting about 150 cm3 of distilled water stained with methylene blue. If the slightest leak appears, the suture is completed.

This check also ensures that there is not a second fistulous orifice, the lack of which would compromise the procedure.

S **The vaginal suture:**

The stitches are passed in BLAIR- DONATI with 3/0 vicryl, to face the vaginal lips to the limits of the detachment so that any dead space between bladder and vagina is eliminated.

The threads are knotted when they have been passed through.

Figure 8, 9 10, 11: Chassar-Moir operation

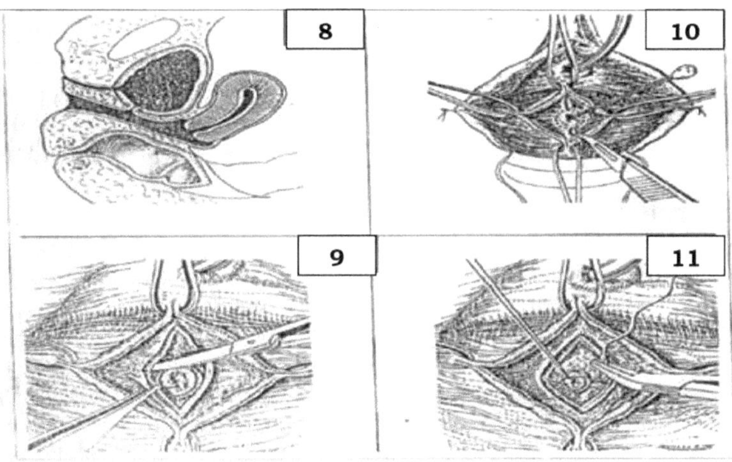

9.3.2.2. Cure of complex fistulas :

The addition of a flap is mandatory in case of attempted closure. Muscle flaps (medial rectus) or MSC flaps (greater lip) may be used.

The procedures are sometimes performed in several stages even in the absence of complications.

Uni- or bilateral episiotomy leading into the ischio-rectal fossae with or without opening the vesico-uterine excavation.

In some situations, the cure of the fistula is impossible. In these cases, palliative treatments are indicated. These include urinary shunts that allow the woman to have a certain comfort:

> Coffey's operation (it consists of a reimplantation of the ureters in the rectum).

> Goodwin's operation (it consists of a ureterosigmoid reimplantation of the two ureters).

> The Bricker operation (this is a transintestinal cutaneous ureterostomy).

> Benchekroun's continental pouch (this is a continental bypass enterocystoplasty known as a continental ileocecal bladder).

9.3.3. Dressing, Monitoring and Post-Operative Nursing Care:

The vagina is then filled gently but completely with wicks soaked in diluted betadine. Within 48 hours, they will contribute to the erasing of dead spaces and the adhesion of tissues.

During the post-operative period, monitoring of the catheter is obviously fundamental. Before the patient can drink abundantly, perfusions and lasix will ensure a good diuresis. This is monitored every hour.

The patient must not be able to pull out her catheter, which is attached to the thigh with a plaster or, better still, to the vulva above the meatus with threads in the first few days. She must also avoid, when she walks, fixing the handle of her bag pipe above the level of her bladder, in order to avoid stagnation or even overpressure at this level.

If the probe stops working and a wash does not restore the situation properly, the probe must be changed.

The probe will be left in place for two weeks.

After removal of the catheter, the first micturition is generally small (100 to 200cc) and usually occurs within three (3) hours if the needs are sufficient. If there is no micturition after 5 to 6 hours, a catheter must be inserted and the quality of the residue must be checked. If the residue is greater than 200cc, the catheter should be left in place for an additional 48 hours (see chapter on complications). Sexual relations are excluded for 1 month after the return of the patient to his home.

9.3.4. Complications and aftermath:

> **Early:** failure of bladder drainage, hemorrhage, wound suppuration, ureteral ligation, endometritis, vulvovaginitis, foreign bodies (compresses).

> **Late:** residual fistulas, sphincter disorders, vaginal sclerosis and atresia, dyspareunia, dysmenorrhea, secondary infertility, etc.

9.3.5. Treatment results:

According to some authors, the results depend on the experience of the operator. For others, the state of the tissues, the etiology as well as the location of the fistula in relation to the bladder neck, condition the prognosis.

90-98% success rate in simple fistulas.

In contrast, success is 45-75% in intermediate and complex fistulas.

III. Methodology:

1-Study framework:

Our study took place in the general surgery department and the FO ward of the Nianankoro Fomba Hospital in Segou.

> Presentation of the general surgery department: it includes two pavilions (male and female surgery) each with: 1 doctor's office, 1 major's office, a treatment room, 4 hospitalization rooms 3ème category with 3 beds in each room (ventilated), 2 VIP rooms 2ème category with 2 beds in each room (ventilated), 2 VIP rooms 1ère category with a bed, an air conditioner, a fan and an internal toilet.

> Presentation of the FO Pavilion: (Reception and accommodation center for women victims of fistula in pre- and post-operation)

It includes: 6 hospitalization rooms with 14 beds, a consultation room, a store, 10 toilets (6 internal and 4 external), a hangar, a laundry room.

> Staff: there are 2 general surgeons, 2 state nurses, 2 nurses, 4 nursing aids, 2 surface agents, one intern.

2- Type and period of study:

This was a prospective, longitudinal study from December 1, 2012 to May 31, 2014, or 18 months.

3-Study population:

These were women with FUGA admitted to the FO ward of the hospital in Segou.

4-Sampling:

2.1- Inclusion criteria:

Our study included patients operated on for obstetric VF and/or AVF during the study period.

2.2- Non-inclusion criteria:

Patients with stress incontinence and non-obstetric urinary fistulas were not included in our study.

5-Variables studied:

S **Socio-demographic aspects:** these concerned age, ethnicity, origin, occupation, marital status, education level, living environment and height.

J **Clinical aspects:** they concerned the reason for consultation, gestational age, parity, age at first marriage, age at first delivery, age at onset of fistula, rank of the causal pregnancy, age of fistula, number of ANC performed, duration of labor, place of delivery, qualifications of the birth attendant, mode of delivery, condition of the child at birth, fistula environment, and type of fistula.

J **Therapeutic aspects: these included** the number of hands, surgical approach, type of anesthesia, technical procedures, and outcome.

6- Data source:

Data were collected from the medical records and from the named survey sheets that we prepared for the study (in the Appendix).

7- Recovery criteria:

We have retained three degrees of recovery:

1st degree: the fistula is closed, without sphincter disturbance, micturition is normal, and no urine leakage.

2nd degree: the fistula is closed, sphincter failure persists with periodic or constant leakage of urine.

3rd degree: the fistula is not closed, it is the failure of the fistula cure.

8-Data collection and analysis:

Data were entered and analyzed on Epi info version 3.5.3 and Microsoft office Word 2007.

IV. Results:

 Sociodemographic aspects :

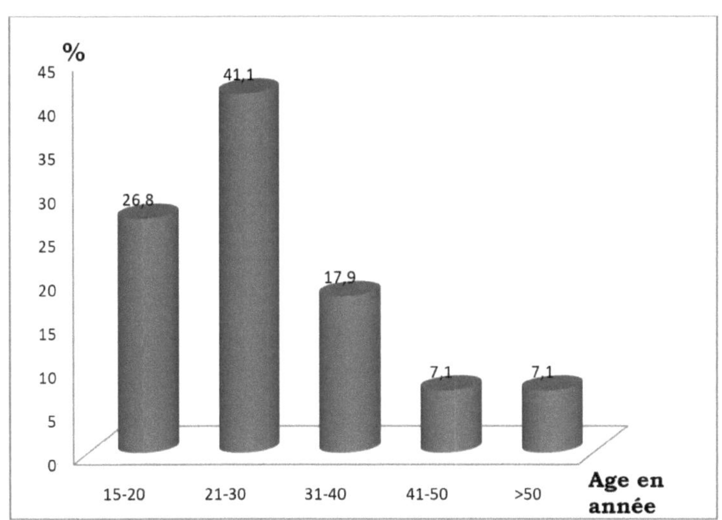

Figure 12: Distribution of patients by age group (year)

Table I: Distribution of patients according to origin

Provenance	Workforce	Percentage
Baraouili	4	7,1
Bla	7	12,5
Outside Ségou* (in French)	9	16,1
Macina	10	17,9
Niono	7	12,5
San	5	8,9
Circle of Segou	**14**	**25,0**
Total	**56**	**100**

*Outside Ségou: Kayes, Sikasso, Gao

Table II: Distribution of patients by occupation

Profession	Workforce	Percentage
Shopkeeper	1	1,8
Housekeeper	**55**	**98,2**
Total	**56**	**100**

Table III: Distribution of patients by marital status

Marital status	Workforce	Percentage
Single	1	1,8
Divorced	5	8,9
Bride	**48**	**85,7**
Widow	2	3,6
Total	**56**	**100**

Table IV: Distribution of Patients by Education Level

Level of education	Workforce	Percentage
Not in school	**54**	**96,4**
Educated	2	3,6
Total	**56**	**100**

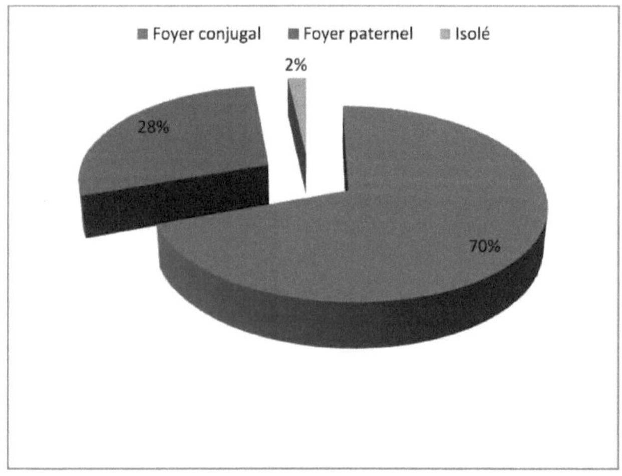

Figure 13: Distribution of patients by living environment

Table V: Distribution of patients by height (in cm)

Size (in cm)	Workforce	Percentage
140-150	12	21,4
151-160	**36**	**64,3**
161-180	8	14,3
Total	**56**	**100**

> **Clinical aspects:**

Table VI: Distribution of patients by reason for consultation

Reason for consultation	Workforce	Percentage
Stool leakage	4	7,1
Urine leakage	**52**	**92,9**
Total	**56**	**100**

Table VII: Distribution of patients by gestational age (number)

Gestité	Workforce	Percentage
1	14	25,0
2	16	28,6
3	3	5,4
>3	**23**	**41,0**
Total	**56**	**100**

Table VIII: Distribution of patients by parity

Parity	Workforce	Percentage
Primipare	**17**	**30,4**
paucipare	16	28,6
Multipare	11	19,6
Large multiparous	12	21,4

Total	56	100

Table IX: Distribution of patients by age at first marriage (in years)

Age at first marriage	Workforce	Percentage
12-20	**51**	**93**
>20	4	7
Total	**55**	**100**

Table X: Distribution of patients by age at first delivery (in years)

Age at first birth	Workforce	Percentage
14-20	**47**	**84**
>20	9	16
Total	**56**	**100**

Table XI: Distribution of patients by age at onset of fistula (year)

Age at onset of fistula	Workforce	percentage
13-20	**23**	**41**
21-30	22	39,3
31-40	9	16,1
>40	2	3,6
Total	**56**	**100**

Table XII: Distribution of patients by rank of causal pregnancy

Rank of the causal pregnancy	Workforce	Percentage
1	**23**	**41,1**
2	12	21,4
3	3	5,4
>3	18	32,1
Total	**56**	**100**

Table XIII: Distribution of patients by age of fistula (in years)

Age of the fistula	Workforce	Percentage
<1	**26**	**46,4**
2-3	12	21,5
4-6	7	12,5
7-10	6	10,7
>10	5	8,9
Total	**56**	**100**

Table XIV: Distribution of patients by number of prenatal visits (ANC) performed

Number of NPCs	Workforce	Percentage
0	**29**	**51,8**
2	5	8,9
3	9	16,1
4	9	16,1
5	3	5,3
6	1	1,8
Total	**56**	**100**

Table XV: Distribution of patients by duration of labor (in hours)

Duration of labor and delivery	Workforce	Percentage
<24	3	5,4
24-72	**37**	**66,1**
>72	16	28,5
Total	**56**	**100**

Table XVI: Distribution of Patients by Place of Delivery of Causal Pregnancy

Place of delivery of the causal pregnancy	Workforce	percentage
Cscom	15	26,8
Csref	**20**	**35,7**

	Workforce	Percentage
Home	11	19,6
Hospital	10	17,9
Total	**56**	**100**

Table XVII: Distribution of Patients by Agent Who Attended Delivery

Assisted delivery by	Workforce	Percentage
Traditional birth attendant	10	17,9
Matron	9	16,1
Physician	**31**	**55,3**
Midwife	6	10,7
Total	**56**	**100**

Table XVIII: Distribution of patients by mode of delivery of the causal pregnancy

Mode of delivery of the causal pregnancy	Workforce	Percentage
Cesarean section	**31**	**55,3**
Instrumental maneuvers	1	1,8
Lower track	24	42,9
Total	**56**	**100**

Table XIX: Distribution of patients according to the child's condition at birth

Condition of the child at birth	Workforce	Percentage
Born dead	**53**	**94,6**
Living	3	5,4
Total	**56**	**100**

Table XX: Distribution of patients by fistula environment

Fistula environment	Workforce	Percentage
Sclerotic	8	14,3
Flexible	**48**	**85,7**
Total	**56**	**100**

Table XXI: Distribution of patients by type of fistula

Type of fistula	Workforce	Percentage
Type I	**17**	**30,4**
Type IIAa	8	14,3
Type IIAb	4	7,1
Type IIAc	1	1,8
Type IIB	4	7,1
Type III	4	7,1
Type IV	2	3,6
Type V	12	21,4
Isolated F.R.V.	4	7,1
Total	**56**	**100**

> **Therapeutic aspects :**

Table XXII: Distribution of patients by number of surgical repairs

Number of surgical repairs	Workforce	Percentage
1	**35**	**62,5**
2	9	16,1
3	4	7,1
4	8	14,3
Total	**56**	**100**

Table XXIII: Distribution of patients by surgical approach

Surgical approach	Workforce	Percentage
Low	**40**	**71,4**
High	15	26,8
Mixed	1	1,8
Total	**56**	**100**

Table XXIV: Distribution of patients by type of anesthesia

Type of anesthesia	Workforce	Percentage
Spinal anesthesia	**56**	**100**
General anesthesia	0	0
Total	**56**	**100**

Table XXV: Distribution of patients according to technical procedures

Technical gestures	Workforce	Percentage
Partial or total cervico-urethral anastomosis	5	9,0
Fistuloraphy + cervico-urethral anastomosis	1	1,8
Fistuloraphy	**46**	**82,1**
Uretroplasty	4	7,1
Total	**56**	**100**

Table XXVI: Distribution of patients by treatment outcome at discharge

Treatment outcome at discharge	Workforce	Percentage
Closed fistula with sphincter disorders	10	17,9
Closed and dried fistula	**35**	**62,5**
Fistula not closed	11	19,6
Total	**56**	**100**

Table XXVII: Distribution of patients by degree of healing according to fistula environment

Guêrison Fistula environment	1er degree	2nd degree	3rd degree	Total
Flexible	32	7	9	48
Sclerotic	3	3	2	8
Total	**35**	**10**	**11**	**56**

Table XVIII: Distribution of patients by degree of healing according to type of fistula

Healing / Type of Fistula	1er degree	2nde degree	3ème degree	Total
Type I	13	1	3	17
Type IIAa	3	4	1	8
Type IIAb	2	1	1	4
Type IIAc	0	0	1	1
Type IIB	0	2	2	4
Type III	4	0	0	4
Type IV	1	1	0	2
Type V	8	1	3	12
Isolated F.R.V.	4	0	0	4
Total	**35**	**10**	**11**	**56**

Table XIX: Distribution of patients according to the degree of recovery by number of surgical repairs

S. Healing / Numbers, hand	1er degree	2nd degree	3rd degree	Total
1st hand	24	5	6	35
2ème hand	6	1	2	9
3ème hand	2	1	1	4
4thme hand	3	3	2	8
Total	**35**	**10**	**11**	**56**

Table XXX: Distribution of patients by degree of healing according to age of fistula

Healing / Age of the	1er degree	2nd degree	3rd degree	Total

fistula				
< 1	19	2	5	26
2-3	8	3	1	12
4-6	5	0	2	7
7-10	2	1	3	6
>10	1	4	0	5
Total	**35**	**10**	**11**	**56**

V. Comments and Discussion:

1- Socio-demographic aspects:

1.1. Age:

The 21 to 30 age group was the most represented (41.1%).

Anoukoum T et al [10] and Dembélé D [11] found respectively 22.4% and 49.2% of patients who were between 20 and 24 years old and 20 and 35 years old.

F.U.G.O. would be frequent in young and active populations; the young age participates in the fetomaternal disproportion in FO.

1.2. Provenance:

All the circles of the Segou region were represented in our series.

The circles of Segou and Macina were predominantly represented with 25% and 17.9% respectively.

Mariko ML [12] and Samaké A [6] found respectively 30% and 23.7% of patients coming from the Macina circle.

Most of the health centers in the Segou circle are managed by obstetric nurses and even matrons in some places.

This may call into question the quality of obstetrical care in these centers.

1.3. Marital status:

The majority of patients were married (85.7%), a rate similar to that found by Samaké A [6]: 84.6%.

This result could be explained by the impact of the husbands' awareness of the possibility of free curative treatment.

1.4. Living Environment:

Patients residing in the marital home were the most represented (69.6%).

This result is similar to that reported by Dembélé D [11] who recorded 53% of patients residing in the marital home. On the other hand, Mariko S [13] and Philippe HJ [14] found respectively 77.8% and 80% of patients isolated.

Today, there is a change in the mentality of the population and fistula patients are more and more accepted.

1.5. Education Level:

Only 3.6% of fistula patients went to school.

Harouna YD et al [15] and Ibrahim et al [16] found respectively 1% and 6% of fistula patients in school.

This would explain why the risk of developing TF exists regardless of education level, but is higher in women with no education.

1.6. Size:

The patients had a height between 151 and 160 cm in 64.3% of cases.

This rate is comparable to those reported by Harouna YD et al [15] and Ouattara S [17] who found respectively 42.3% and 86.2% of women with a height below 160 cm.

Short stature would constitute a real risk factor for the occurrence of FM. Mensah A. [18] finds that this factor does not play a predominant role insofar as 70% of his patients are over 20 years of age and 50% are multiparous. He blames the lack of surveillance of pregnancies and deliveries on the under-medicalization of the rural world.

2-Clinical aspects:

2.1. Reason for consultation:

Fifty-two (92.9%) of the women consulted for involuntary urine loss versus 7.1% who consulted for vaginal stool loss.

In most cases, TF is genitourinary, as confirmed by several previous studies in which the loss of urine, as reported by the patient herself, was the main reason for consultation [16, 19, 20].

2.2. Parity and causal pregnancy:

Primiparous women were the most represented (30.4%) compared to 19.6% of multiparous women.

Bouya P.A et al [21] found 38% of primiparous and 15% of multiparous.

While primiparous and large multiparous women are at risk for fistula and incontinence, the causes are different.

- For primiparous females, the immaturity of the pelvis is the cause.

- For large multiparous females, the cause is usually dynamic.

The uterus and the pelvic floor, having been too often solicited, get tired and one often observes a stop of the labor of childbirth.

2.3. Age at first marriage, first delivery, and onset of fistula:

Fifty-one of the 55 married patients (93%) were married before 20 years of age, and 47 of the 56 patients (84%) gave birth for the first time under 20 years of age.

Before the age of 20, 41% of patients started their suffering in the urine with the appearance of the fistula.

This can be explained by the persistence in our societies of early marriage of young girls with immature pelvis, source of mechanical dystocia by fetomaternal disproportion.

2.4. Age of fistula:

The majority of patients (46.4%) were operated on within one year of the onset of the fistula. This rate is lower than that reported by Coulibaly M [22] who found 60%.

This rate can be explained by the impact of the population's awareness of the free and available management of FM.

2.5. Number of ANCs performed :

Twenty-nine (51.8%) of the patients did not undergo ANC, a rate lower than those reported by Ouattara S [17] and Dembélé D [11] who found respectively 85% and 70.5% of women who did not undergo ANC. This can be explained by the lack of financial resources for travel and the cost of ANC.

The ANCs did not allow 27 of our patients to escape from F.U.G.O. This would call into question the quality of these ANCs.

2.6. Duration of labor:

Patients who delivered between 24 and 72 hours of labor were the most represented (66.1%). This rate is similar to that of Dembélé D [11] who found 66.7%.

It is lower than those of Berthé H [23] and Koïta A.K [24] who reported 75% and

93.94% respectively.

This may be due to a lack of information about pregnancy, as many women attempt to give birth at home without difficulty and return to the health centers late.

However, long labor does not only explain the occurrence of fistula.

2.7. Place of delivery of the causal pregnancy:

Patients who gave birth in a health facility were the most represented (80.4%) compared to 19.6% of women who gave birth at home.

This rate is similar to that reported by Coulibaly M [22] who found 74.3%.

This could be explained by the recent increase in the number of health centers throughout the country and the fact that the majority of parturients arrived with the process of fistulization already underway due to the length of the labor period.

2.8. Qualification of the deliverer and the mode of delivery of the causal pregnancy :

Thirty-one (55.3%) of deliveries were assisted by doctors; on the other hand, Ouattara S [17] reported in his study: 52.1% of deliveries assisted by matrons.

The majority of women (55.3%) delivered by cesarean section.

The doctors performed a caesarean section for maternal rescue with the process of fistulization already underway given the predominance of low fistulas in our series.

2.9. Child's condition at birth:

Fifty-three (94.6%) of the women lost their child during the delivery that generated the fistula, it agrees with that of Mensah A and Coll [18]: 96%.

This high mortality is explained by poor monitoring of pregnancies and unassisted labor.

3-Classification of obstetric fistula:

For this we used the classification of the urology service of the CHU of Point "G" (Pr Ouattara Kalilou et al) [5].

3.1. Fistula environment:

Forty-eight (85.7%) of the fistulas were located in a soft vagina; this rate is comparable to that found by Samaké A [6]: 70%.

This result can be explained by the early management of fistulas because of the flexibility of the vagina, which is a guarantee of successful surgical treatment.

3.2. TF Type:

All types of fistulas were represented in our series.

Vesico-vaginal septum fistula was the most represented (30.4%). It is lower than that of Anoukoum T et al [10]: 80.98%.

Four cases (7.1%) of isolated recto-vaginal fistula were identified.

4-Therapeutic aspects:

4.1. Number of surgical repairs:

First-hand fistulas were the most represented (62.5%).

It is lower than that of Ouattara S [17]: 39%.

4.2. Surgical approach:

This result is similar to that reported by Moudouni S et al [20] who found 70%.

The vaginal route was for us the best route, because it is the most anatomical and the simplest, offering a perfect exposure of the type of FO most represented in our series. It can be used even in the case of vaginal sclerosis thanks to enlargement devices such as episiotomy.

4.3. Type of anesthesia:

All our operations were performed under spinal anesthesia because of the simplicity of the technique and the motor block responsible for a good muscle relaxation facilitating exposure and surgical maneuvers.

Spinal anesthesia avoided the risks of general anesthesia.

4.4. Technical gestures:

Fistuloraphy, inspired by the Chassar-Moir technique, was the most common procedure in our series (82.1%). It is higher than that found by Steg A [25]: 68.9%.

The choice of technical procedures depends on the fistula environment and the type of fistula.

4.5. Treatment outcomes at discharge:

In our series, we recorded 35 cases of closed and dried fistulas with 62.5% and 10 cases of closed fistulas with sphincter disorders which could be explained by sphincter insufficiency caused by obstetrical trauma.

In 11 patients, the fistula was not closed, even though the urine leakage was considerably reduced with or without retention of micturition: this is a failure of the fistula cure.

Elsewhere, cure rates are high: 86% in the series by Mensah A et al in Senegal [18], 91% in the series by Perata in Kenya [26] and 65.1% in the series by Dembélé D [11].

The success of the surgical treatment depends on many factors:

• **Fistula environment:** Of the 35 closed and dried fistulas, 31 were located in a soft vagina.

• **Type of fistula:** The majority of closed and dried fistulas (13 cases) were vesico-vaginal septum fistulas.

• **Number of surgical repairs:** First-hand fistulas were in the majority with 24 cases out of 35 closed and dried fistulas.

• **Age of the fistula:** Fistulas less than one year old were in the majority with 19 cases out of 35 closed and dried fistulas.

Our result is similar to that reported by Tembély A et al [27] who found 212 healed fistulas out of 300 operated, among which 143 were fistulas of the vesico-vaginal septum located on a soft vagina.

This result leads us to conclude that fistulas of the vesicovaginal septum located on a soft vagina, operated for the first time within one year of appearance, offer a good therapeutic result.

Nevertheless, the chances of recovery would be low but not zero for other types of fistulas up to 4 interventions.

VI. Conclusion:

The F.U.G.O remains a real public health problem in our region despite the efforts made in the fight against this plague.

It is a pathology of young women that affects all socio-professional groups. It reflects the inaccessibility of parturients to health services: availability of qualified agents, lack of financial means and the geographical location of health facilities.

The success of the surgical treatment is conditioned by the importance of the urogenital lesions (vaginal sclerosis, type of fistula, number of repair attempts, age of the fistula).

In spite of the successes recorded in the surgical management of this scourge, its eradication requires the application of preventive measures such as: the monitoring of pregnancies by ANCs, the monitoring of labor and delivery practices by qualified health care personnel, the instruction and education of the population in health, but also the social integration of women victims who have undergone surgery and have recovered.

Recommendations:

At the end of our study we made the following recommendations:

> **To the political authorities**

J Sustained enrollment of girls

Training and availability of health workers to ensure quality obstetrical care at all levels of health care, especially in the countryside

J Free prenatal care.

J Improved and free transportation for women in labour.

J Socioeconomic integration of women healed of fistula.

> **To the social and health care personnel**

Raising women's awareness so that they attend health centers for regular prenatal consultations and give birth in a specialized environment

J Raising awareness of the harms of early marriage

Awareness of traditional birth attendants to evacuate parturients as soon as the duration of labor reaches 6 hours.

> **To the public**

J Sustained enrollment of girls

J Encouraging parturients to attend health centers to monitor their pregnancies until delivery

J Avoidance of early marriage.

Bibliographic references:

1. WHO Regional Office for Africa, Reproductive Health. Health Information Files for the WHO African Region. AFR/INF/99-1.

2. UNFPA. The second meeting of the working group for the prevention and treatment of obstetric fistula, Addis Ababa, 31 October-1 November 2002.

3. Labarrère A et al. Obstetric urogenital fistula: about two observations in France. Gynécologie Obstétrique & Fertilité .2011 ;39:328- 331.

4. DNS/DSR. Situational analysis of SONU structures; Bamako; 2008.

5. Ouattara K. First congress of ACAF, the vesico-vaginal fistula: a public health problem; December 7-8-9; Bamako; 2005.

6. Samaké A. Epidemiological study of obstetrical vesico-vaginal fistulas at the Nianankoro Fomba Hospital in Segou, Mali, in 52 cases [Thesis: Medicine]. [Bamako: FMPOS; 2010

7. Camey M. Les fistules obstétricales, Progrès en urologie 7, Bd, Flandrin-75116 Paris, 4éme trimestre 1998, 328 pages.

8. Rouviere. Human anatomy: descriptive and topographic. Volume II, Masson et Cie 1970, Bd Saint Germain- Paris- 1970.

9. Kamina P. Anatomie gynécologique et obstétricale ; 3éme édition remaniée, Paris, Maloine, 1979.

10. Anoukoum T et al. Epidemiological, etiological and therapeutic aspects of obstetric fistula in Togo. Progrès en urologie.2010; 20 :71-76.

11. Dembélé D. Campaigns for the Management of Vesico-Vaginal Fistula in the Urology Service of the Point G University Hospital. [Bamako: FMPOS; 2010.

12. Mariko ML. Study of obstetrical vesico-vaginal fistulas at the NianankoroFomba hospital in Segou, about 30 cases. [Bamako: FMPOS; 2006.

13. Mariko S. Les fistules uro-génitales : expérience du service d'urologie de l'hôpital du Point G à propos de 72 cas. [Bamako: FMPOS; 2000.

14. Phillipe H J, Goffine F, Janckrye, Traore B. Obstetrical fistulas. Encycl. Med Chir (Elsevier, Paris), obstetrics.1998, 7P.

15. **Harouna YD et al.** Vesico-vaginal fistula of obstetrical cause.Médecine d'Afrique Noire .2001 ;48 (2) :55-9.

16. **Ibrahim T, Sadiq AU, Daniel SO.** Characteristics of VVF patients as seen at the specialist hospital.West Afr. J. Med. 2000;19 (1):59-63.

17. **Ouattara S.** Problem of the treatment of VVF in Mali: 94 cases. [Bamako: FMPOS; 2004.

18. **Mensah A, Diagne B.A.** Les fistules vésico-vaginales, aspects étiopathogéniques et thérapeutiques au Sénégal.J. Urol.1992 ;98(3) :148- 151.

19. **Ouattara K, Traore ML, Cisse C.** Some statistical aspects of vesico-vaginal fistula in the Republic of Mali. About 134 cases. Médecine d'Afrique Noire.1991;38(12):856-860.

20. **Moudouni S et al.** Obstetric vesico-vaginal fistulas. About 114 cases. Progrès en Urologie.2001 ;11 :103-108.

21. **Bouya PA et al.** Retrospective study of 34 urogenital fistulas of obstetric origin. Gynécologie Obstétrique & Fertilité.2002 ;30 :780-783.

22. **Coulibaly M.** Étude des fistules vésico-vaginales obstétricales à l'hôpital Niankoro Fomba de Ségou. [Bamako: FMPOS; 2009.

23. **BerthéH.** L'étude des fistules uro-génitales dans le service d'urologie de l'hôpital Nianankoro Fomba de Ségou à propos de 16 cas. [Bamako: FMPOS; 1999.

24. **Koïta A.K.** Quelques aspects des fistules vésico-vaginales observées à l'hôpital du Point G. [Bamako: ENMP; 1983.

25. **Steg A, P. Vialatte, Olivier C.** The treatment of vesico- vaginal fistulas by the Chassar-Moir technique. Journal urologie.1997 ; 11(2) :103-107.

26. **Lufuma LN, Tschipeta N, Uwonda A, Tozin B.** African obstetric vesicovaginal fistulas. About fifty seven cases.Ann Urol.1985;19(2):87-9.

27. **Tembely A et al.** Contribution to the classification of obstetric vesicovaginal fistula. Mali Médical.2009; 24(2) :50-2.

APPENDICES

DATA SHEET

Name : Koné

First Name : Mahamadou Abdoulaye

Email : Konemahamadou35@yahoo.fr

Tel: 63195619/75117450

Title of the thesis: Obstetrical urogenital fistulas at the Nianankoro Fomba Hospital in Segou, about 56 cases.

Academic year: 2014-2015

City of defense: Bamako

Country of origin: Republic of Mali.

Place of deposit: Library of the Faculty of Medicine and Odontostomatology of Bamako. BP : 1805

Area of interest: Urology, Gyneco-obstetrics.

Abstract: This was a prospective and longitudinal study of 18 months (1er December 2012 to May 31, 2014), which took place in the department of general surgery and the obstetric fistula pavilion of the Nianankoro Fomba Hospital of Segou on the management of 56 cases of obstetric urogenital fistulas. Our study had the following objectives: General:

> Studying obstetrical urogenital fistulas at the Nianankoro Fomba Hospital in Segou

Specific:

> Analyze the socio-demographic aspects

> Identify risk factors

> Analyze the therapeutic aspects

Tench aged 21 to 30 years were the most represented with 41.1%.

41% of patients contracted fistula before the age of 20. The circle of Segou provided 25% of the sample. 64.3% of the patients had a height between 151-160 centimeters. The living environment was conjugal in 69.6% of cases, and the majority of patients were housewives.

Primiparous women, with 30.4%, paid the highest price for the disability. Fistulas less than one year old constituted 46.4% of the sample. 51.8% of the patients had not benefited from prenatal consultations. 66.1% suffered from a long labor of 24 to 72 hours.

80.4% of patients gave birth in a health facility, Caesarean section was the mode of delivery in 55.3% of cases and resulted in stillbirth in 94.6% of cases. The delivery was assisted by doctors in 55.3% of cases. The reason for consultation was urinary loss in 92.9% of cases. The fistula was type I in 30.4% of the cases, located in a soft vagina in 85.7% of the cases. 62.5% of the patients were at their first attempt of surgical repair.

All our patients were operated under spinal anesthesia. The vaginal route was the most used with 71.4%. Fistulorraphy inspired by the Chassar-Moir technique was preferred. 62.5% of the fistulas were closed and dried.

Key words: obstetric urogenital fistula, epidemiology, treatment.

SURVEY FORM

<u>Socio-demographic aspects:</u>

Q1- Registration no:

Q2- Name:

Q3- First name:

Q4- Age:

Q5-Ethnia

Q6- Provenance:

Q7-Profession:

Q8-Marital status: <u>I I</u>

1. married 2.divorced 3.single 4.widowed

Q9-Level of education: _______ | |

1. literate 2.illiterate

Q10-Living environment: I_I

1. Maternal home 2.Paternal home 3.Foster home 4.Isolated

Q11- Size:

<u>Clinical aspects:</u>

Q12-reason for consultation: □

1. Leakage of urine 2.leakage of stool 3.leakage of urine and stool

Q13-Age at first marriage:

Q14-Age at first delivery:

Q15-Age at time of fistula onset:

Q16-Rank of causal pregnancy:

Q17-Age of fistula (in years):

Q18-Was the pregnancy desired? □

1. Yes 2.no

Q19-Number of prenatal visits (ANC)

Q20-What was the duration of labor in the causal pregnancy (in hours):

Q21-Place of delivery of the causal pregnancy: I_I

1. Home 2.Cscom 3.Csref 4.Hospital

Q22-Was the delivery assisted? Yes □ No □

If yes by whom? Physician □Nurse □Midwife □Matron □ Q23-Mode of delivery of causal pregnancy: I_I

1. 2.instrumental maneuvers 3.cesarean section

Q24-Child's condition at birth: I_I_I

1. Alive 2.stillborn

Q25-Menstruation? I_I

1. Yes 2.no

Q26-Environment of the fistula:l

1. Fistula on soft vagina 2.fistula on sclerotic vagina

Q27-Type of fistula: I I

2. Type I: Vesico-vaginal septum fistula

3. Type IIAa: Cervicourethrovaginal fistula without destruction of the urethra

4. Type IIAb : Partial cervico-urethral disinsertion

5. Type IIAc : Total cervico-urethral disinsertion

6. Type IIB: Cervicourethrovaginal fistula with destruction of the urethra

7. Type III: Trigono-cervico-utero-vaginal fistulas

8. Type VI: Complex (mixed) fistulas

9. Type V : High fistulas (retrotrigonal)

10. Isolated recto-vaginal fistula

11. LIF + LIF

Therapeutic aspects:

Q28-Number of hands I

Q29-Surgical approach: _____________ I I

1. Low 2.High 3.Mixed

Q30-Type of anesthesia: I I

1. Spinal anesthesia 2. General anesthesia 3. combined anesthesia Q31- Technical procedures: I I

1.fistuloraphy (FVV, FRV)

2. Urethroplasty (neo urethra)

3. Partial or total cervico-urethral anastomosis

4. Uretero - bladder reimplantation

5. Vaginal plasty + or - cervical deflation

6. Urinary diversion (Goowing, Bricker, Coffey, Kock or Benchekroun continental pouch)

7. Other :

Q32- Outcome of the treatment: I I

1. Closed and dried fistula

2. Closed fistula with sphincter disorders (incontinence)

3. Fistula not closed

HIPPOCRATIC OATH

In the presence of the masters of this faculty, of my dear fellow students, before the effigy of Hippocrates, I promise and swear, in the name of the Supreme Being, to be faithful to the laws of honor and probity in the practice of medicine.

I will give my free care to the needy and will never demand a salary above my work, I will not participate in any clandestine sharing of fees.

My eyes shall not see what goes on inside the houses, my tongue shall not speak of the secrets that are entrusted to me, and my state shall not be used to corrupt morals, nor to promote crime.

I will not allow considerations of religion, nation, race, party or class to come between my duty and my patient.

I will maintain absolute respect for human life from the moment of conception.

Even under threat, I will not admit to use my medical knowledge against the laws of humanity.

Respectful and grateful to my teachers, I will give back to their children the education I received from their fathers.

May men give me their esteem if I am faithful to my promises.

May I be covered with opprobrium and despised by my colleagues if I fail to do so.

I swear!

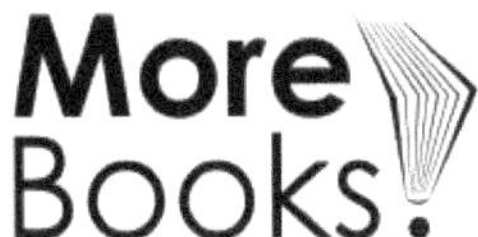

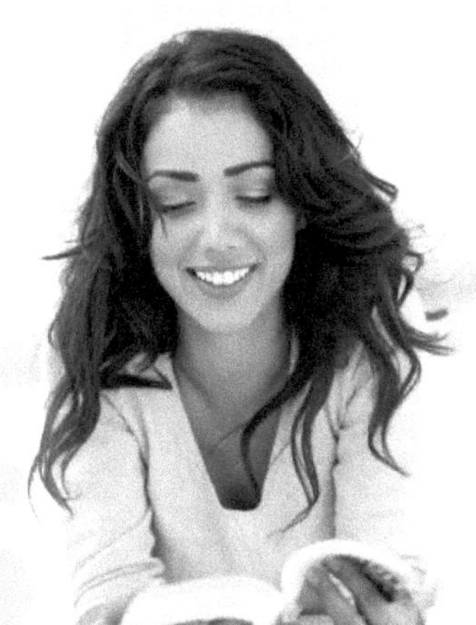

I want morebooks!

Buy your books fast and straightforward online - at one of world's fastest growing online book stores! Environmentally sound due to Print-on-Demand technologies.

Buy your books online at
www.morebooks.shop

Kaufen Sie Ihre Bücher schnell und unkompliziert online – auf einer der am schnellsten wachsenden Buchhandelsplattformen weltweit! Dank Print-On-Demand umwelt- und ressourcenschonend produziert.

Bücher schneller online kaufen
www.morebooks.shop

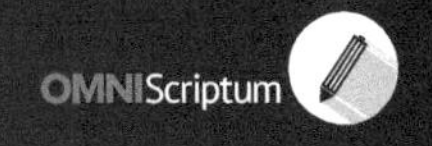